About the author

Peggy Brusseau is an experienced fitness instructor who
gives regular classes and lectures on using movement to
relieve pain and improve overall well-being and mobility.
Her sound knowledge of herbal medicine was acquired
when she ran a small-holding, with its own herb garden.
She has appeared frequently on television and radio to
talk about the importance of fitness, health and diet.

A WI HELP YOURSELF GUIDE

Overcoming Rheumatism and Arthritis Naturally

Peggy Brusseau

CENTURY

LONDON · MELBOURNE · AUCKLAND · JOHANNESBURG

Important Note

All the therapies described in this book have one thing in common –
that is, they have been reported as giving some degree of
symptomatic relief from rheumatism for some people. Just as there
are many types of rheumatism, so there are many possible lines of
treatment – some effective, some less so. If you suffer from a
rheumatic disease, you should always seek qualified medical
treatment, and you should not attempt self-treatment with any of the
therapies outlined in this book without first discussing and agreeing
the proposed treatment with your doctor. Diagnosis and treatment
of medical conditions is a responsibility shared between you and
your doctor, and neither the author nor publisher of this book can
accept responsibility for the consequences of treatment with
therapies described herein.

Copyright © Peggy Brusseau 1988

All rights reserved

First published in 1988 by Century Hutchinson Ltd
Brookmount House, 62–65 Chandos Place, London WC2N 4NW

Century Hutchinson Australia (Pty) Ltd
PO Box 496, 16–22 Church Street, Hawthorn,
Victoria 3122, Australia

Century Hutchinson New Zealand Ltd
PO Box 40–086, 32–34 View Road, Glenfield,
Auckland 10, New Zealand

Century Hutchinson South Africa (Pty) Ltd
PO Box 337, Bergvlei 2012, South Africa

Photoset in 9pt Sabon (Linotron 202)
by Deltatype Lecru, Ellesmere Port, Cheshire

Printed and bound in Great Britain by
Mackays of Chatham

British Library Cataloguing in Publication Data

Brusseau, Peggy
  Overcoming rheumatism and arthritis
  naturally.—(A WI help-yourself guide).
  1. Arthritis   2. Rheumatism
  3. Naturopathy
  I. Title   II. Series
  616.7'2065   RC933

ISBN 0–7126–1981–X

CONTENTS

1

RHEUMATISM AND ARTHRITIS: EVERYBODY'S HEARTACHE

You are not alone. More than eight million people in Britain suffer from a rheumatic disease. With more than 200 rheumatic diseases to choose from that may not be surprising, but it is a heartache. These diseases take strength, mobility and happiness from each person who suffers from them, and it has been so for thousands of years. Why, it seems that even the dinosaurs suffered from this scourge!

The rheumatic diseases affect us all – young and old, fit and disabled, male and female – because rheumatism and arthritis can appear at any age in just about any person. And even if you don't suffer yourself, you probably know and care for someone who does.

For a variety of reasons, some not yet known, in rheumatic disease the tissues in and around the joints of the body begin to alter and create distressing symptoms. These include pain, stiffness, inflammation, deformity and even total joint destruction. In some diseases few joints are affected, while in other forms it seems that the whole body has turned against itself so that no joint is left unharmed.

Furthermore, for every answer that is found regarding their cause and cure, another question seems to appear in its place. The rheumatic diseases, with the exception of gout and rheumatic fever, are virtually unchallenged in the power they wield. Many treatments have been derived which minimize the effect of disease, once it has struck. But no treatment has been manufactured which can prevent rheumatic disease or cure you of its consequences. No treatment, except one.

The rheumatic diseases can be prevented and cured by health. The reason they appear in the first place is that the body is not in good condition. In other words, they are caused by illness.

Before you throw down the book in disgust, consider for a moment that the rheumatic diseases rarely kill. They erode. They erode your previous good health, your strength, agility, and pain-free ability to move. Yet who can say when that erosion began?

It is highly probable that the erosion of your health began months or even years before the first symptoms of rheumatic disease became obvious. It is also probable that, at some point before the symptoms appeared, you were unknowingly in a position to *prevent* them occurring. Your diet, environment, level of stress, attitude or any number of other activities or characteristics which belonged to you almost certainly began a silent illness which eventually caused or contributed to your current rheumatic disease.

This book is about health. However ill you are, however disillusioned and riddled with pain, you can still regain some of the health which you have lost. Health is what every part of you wants and it can be regained in some measure by retracing your steps and correcting the way in which you fulfil your basic needs – from eating and sleeping to walking and thinking.

There are three simple steps towards this end – the three A's of health.

1) Keep a good **attitude** – decide that you *really* want to be well (some people don't, you know!) and that you will do what you can to achieve the best health possible for you.

2) Learn the **alternatives** which are open to you – can you change your diet, your mattress and your morning routine to improve your lot, even if you can't change your lower spine?

3) Then do it! Real benefits come from **action** – let your new attitude help you to *use* the health-giving alternatives you have found.

Hopefully, this book will get you started. It is necessarily brief on each of the topics it introduces. If you can, read through all of it in order to get an outline picture of the rheumatic diseases and the great number of treatments available for you to choose from. Then, do what you can to help yourself to health!

Rheumatism in particular

● Rheumatism is a very general term which is used to help describe a great many disorders. In order for a condition to be rheumatic, it must involve inflammation, degeneration or metabolic disturbance of joints, muscles, bursae, tendons, ligaments, or connective tissues. Pain, stiffness and limited movement in the joints and muscles are the most noticeable symptoms of rheumatism, and most of us suffer, at some point in our lives, from symptoms which are included in this definition. In many cases, these symptoms are due to injury, strain or fatigue rather than the beginnings of a rheumatic disease. Therefore, it is important to discover the cause of any symptoms so that appropriate treatment may be sought.

● Anyone can suffer from rheumatism, no matter how young, old or otherwise healthy you are, but some people are more vulnerable to certain forms of it than others. For instance, rheumatic fever, an acute form of rheumatism, attacks children and adolescents, while rheumatoid arthritis prefers women between 20 and 45 years of age. Infection and hormonal changes trigger some forms of rheumatism but the cause of other forms is still unknown.

● If you suffer from general aches and pains, you might simply complain about your 'rheumatics' and leave it at that. However, if the suffering continues, or becomes worse, you should visit your GP who will explore your symptoms and medical history with you. He or she will diagnose your problem and recommend treatment.

● Note the name your doctor gives to your condition as well as the treatment recommended and read through the appropriate sections of this book. In the section headed 'What's Your Problem?', specific disorders are discussed and their various names listed. All of these disorders have symptoms which place them under the very broad heading of rheumatism.

Arthritis in particular
● Arthritis is a form of rheumatism which is suffered in the joints and connective tissue. Whereas rheumatism can affect a variety of tissue, arthritis affects only the joints and connective tissue.

There are two main types of arthritis: inflammatory and non-inflammatory. Inflammatory arthritis is either apparent or non-apparent. Just as it sounds, apparent inflammation means you can see it: the inflamed area goes warm, red and swollen and probably feels painful. Non-apparent inflammation means you cannot see it, though changes in your blood indicate that inflammation is occurring.

Non-inflammatory arthritis tends to concentrate on degeneration of the joint, as in osteoarthritis. You will still feel pain and loss of mobility, but there will be no inflammation, apparent or otherwise.

● Arthritis has many forms and, like rheumatism, can affect anyone. While some types are caused by trauma, infection or metabolic changes, other types are part of ageing *for some people*. There are further types out of the more than 100 different arthritic disorders whose cause is unknown.

CROSS-SECTION OF A JOINT

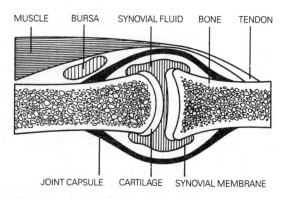

MUSCLE BURSA SYNOVIAL FLUID BONE TENDON

JOINT CAPSULE CARTILAGE SYNOVIAL MEMBRANE

● If you feel your symptoms are centred around your joints then a visit to your GP is a good idea. He or she will discuss your symptoms with you, as well as your medical history. If a diagnosis of arthritis is made, it will probably have a more specific name and may or may not actually include the word 'arthritis'. Learn as much as you can from this visit, including how your GP expects the disease to progress. You will need this information in order to choose the most successful treatment for your condition.

Before we go on, take a look at this diagram of a joint. You will see the tissues in and around the joint which are mentioned in the disease descriptions which follow.

What's your problem?

Ankylosing Spondylitis

● This form of ankylosis affects the spine. It is an inflammatory condition, also called Bekhterev's disease or Marie-Struempell disease, which usually starts in the joints of the lower back and pelvis.

● Ankylosing spondylitis begins with inflammation of the tissues in and around your spine. The inflammation causes pain and stiffness which leads, eventually, to loss of mobility. Loss of mobility, in turn, affects the progress of your disease. Calcium gradually deposits in the muscles and ligaments around your spine, your pain and stiffness increases and fibrous tissue and cartilage may even be converted into bony tissue. These developments further reduce your mobility and, in some cases, the complication of osteoporosis of the spine may follow. A vicious cycle is established and by the time true ankylosis – complete union of the joints – occurs, a great deal of mobility has been lost and significant tissue changes have taken place.

● Ankylosing spondylitis moves progressively up from the pelvis and lower back to include the middle and upper spine and the neck. The hips and the joints between the ribs can also be affected and in this case breathing becomes more difficult.

● Young men number highest in those affected by ankylosing spondylitis and their symptoms are usually as just described. In women, however, the pain, inflammation and stiffness usually begin in the neck rather than the lower back and pelvis. The cause of this disease is unknown. However, a tissue type (HLA B27) is present in 90–95% of sufferers therefore it is, in part, considered an hereditary disease.

● A strong and determined outlook is essential to deal with ankylosing spondylitis. A certain amount of pain will need to be tolerated, exercise taken when possible and some thought given to the home and working environments. For instance, sleeping on a firm mattress will help prevent deformation of the spine and chairs should be selected which give support to the lower back especially.

If it is allowed to go un-arrested, severe disability may result from this disease. Your initial task must be to reduce pain so that mobility may be maintained for as long as possible. Oddly, pain relief can usually be achieved if you keep the area immobile until pain and inflammation are reduced – *then* improve your mobility. In the short term, a splint can be used to keep a joint immobile, or non-steroidal anti-inflammatory drugs, and in some cases radiotherapy, may be used to relieve pain. Then, physiotherapy may be performed to maintain or improve mobility. In severe cases, hospital treatment and the use of very powerful anti-inflammatory drugs, such as Phenylbutazone, may be recommended by your doctor.

● Natural remedies: Exercise (chapter 5), Hands On and Lifestyle (chapter 6).

Ankylosis

● In this disorder, the joint is made completely immobile because it actually grows together due to excess production of bone cells. A 'false' ankylosis also exists in which fibrous tissue (similar to the tissue of a ligament) is produced in excess, instead of bone, and results in greatly reduced mobility of a joint. These terms are often used inter-changeably but they have very different underlying conditions.

Ankylosis rarely exists on its own – another form of arthritis generally precedes it. For instance, those who have severe rheumatoid arthritis in the spine often suffer ankylosis of some parts of the spine or pelvis. The inflam-mation and consequent destruction of the joints and sur-rounding tissue create conditions in the joint which allow ankylosis to occur. This process is painful in its initial stages, but once the ankylosis is complete there is little or no pain, though mobility is greatly reduced.

● Ankylosis of a joint is sometimes induced through surgery where a 'pin' is used to fix a joint into an immovable position. Bone growth is then encouraged within the joint to confirm the ankylosis. This operation is used very success-fully in some cases of osteoarthritis where degeneration in the joint is at a very advanced stage. While pain is usually eliminated by this surgery, the other, movable joints are made to work harder and it is important to build strength and correct posture to protect them.

● Natural remedies: Hands On and Lifestyle (chapter 6).

Bursitis

● You have no doubt heard of 'housemaid's knee' and 'tennis elbow', but have you ever heard of 'policemen's heel', 'miner's elbow' or 'weaver's bottom'? These are all forms of bursitis, an inflammatory condition of the bursae.

Bursae are small, fluid-filled sacs which lie between bones, joints, muscles and tendons. They are there to reduce friction between these tissues and so make your movements easier and more comfortable. An inflamed bursa will cause pain and swelling in the surrounding area and will make it difficult for you to move that part of your body.

● Bursitis can affect anyone of any age. It is known for reflecting your work and your way of life, as the common names for it prove. Generally, inflammation of the bursae is caused when you repeat one movement too often or too strenuously, as in tennis elbow, or by placing too much pressure on one area or joint, as in housemaid's knee. Bursitis can also be caused by shoes that pinch or rub or by a sharp blow to one joint. In these cases the small sacs become inflamed in an attempt to reduce friction in the affected area.

Occasionally, calcium deposits in nearby tendons will irritate the bursae, causing a great deal of pain and inflammation. This is especially common in the shoulder region and certain movements, such as pulling on your coat, become very difficult. The calcium deposits often dissolve of their own accord within about a fortnight (see Tendinitis). An X-ray is sometimes used to determine the cause of pain and stiffness if bursitis is not obviously the cause.

● When bursitis occurs you should immediately rest the affected area by altering your movements, or removing the cause of irritation, such as a poor-fitting shoe. Use of an ice-pack helps to reduce the initial swelling. Non-steroidal anti-inflammatory drugs are used to relieve pain and, in severe cases, surgical removal of calcium deposits is indicated. Exercise or physiotherapy is essential for complete recovery after surgery.

● Natural remedies: Homoeopathy & Biochemics (chapter 7), Plants (chapter 8), and From the East (chapter 11).

Climactic Arthritis SEE Menopausal Arthritis

Dry Joint

● This form of rheumatoid arthritis is also called chronic villous arthritis. Its symptoms include squeaky or cracking joints, especially of the knee, and generally impaired function of the affected joint.

● The synovial membrane produces excess tissue which grows into the joint cavity. The synovial fluid is displaced and inflammation follows, causing painful and reduced movement.

● Orthodox treatment usually involves the use of anti-inflammatory analgesics or non-steroidal anti-inflammatory drugs.

● Natural remedies: Supplements (chapter 4), Homoeopathy & Biochemics (chapter 7), and Water (chapter 10).

False Ankylosis SEE Ankylosis

Fibrositis

● Also called muscular rheumatism, rheumatoid myositis and fibrofascitis, this inflammatory ailment affects the white, fibrous tissue of your body.

● Pain, stiffness and depression accompany the inflammation, which is caused by an over-production of the cells which make up muscle sheaths, fascia and other fibrous and connective tissue. The pain and stiffness of fibrositis are suffered in muscles and tendons. Anyone may suffer this disorder, which may appear and disappear quite suddenly.

● Heat treatments, physiotherapy and anti-inflammatory analgesics are among the orthodox treatments.

● Natural remedies: Supplements (chapter 4), Exercise (chapter 5), Hands On and Lifestyle (chapter 6), Homoeopathy & Biochemics (chapter 7), Plants (chapter 8), Water (chapter 10), and From the East (chapter 11).

Gonococcal Arthritis SEE Infective Arthritis

Gout

● Gout is a metabolic disorder which allows an excess of uric acid to accumulate in the body, causing urate crystals to form. Some of these crystals form into hard lumps, called 'tophi', which appear in the ear lobe or in and around a joint. More crystals may collect in the kidneys, where they cause damage, or may even form into stones.

If you have gout, you are afflicted with very acute attacks of arthritis. These are due to the urate crystal deposits causing damage to your joints. The first of these attacks comes on suddenly, often at night, though you may have previously felt very healthy. A small joint, usually of the big toe, is the first joint to be affected. It becomes very red, shiny and swollen and is exceptionally tender. In gout, the pain feels more on the surface and much sharper than in other forms of arthritis, so that often it is unbearable to have the area around the joint even touched. Other symptoms include a high temperature, possibly constipation and a feeling of nausea.

After the first acute attack, gout may become a chronic – regularly occurring – disorder. The symptoms may increase in frequency and duration, though not necessarily in their intensity. Instead the disease may become more general, with more joints becoming arthritic through damage by the 'tophi', or urate crystals. This stage of the disease is sometimes called 'gouty arthritis'.

● Only about one in twenty gout sufferers is a woman; the other 95 per cent are men in middle age. The error in metabolism which causes gout is thought to be inherited in most cases, although damaged or diseased kidneys may cause it in some. The aged belief that gout is caused by eating and drinking in excess is not strictly true, although excesses may aggravate the disorder in those who are predisposed to it.

● Treatment begins with rest and pain relief. Do not take aspirin during an attack of gout as it can block the passage of uric acid and make the pain worse. Prescription-only drugs are available for relief of pain and symptoms, for instance:

Colchicine, a drug made from a crocus, has been in use for hundreds of years to relieve the pain and inflammation of gout. It can, in some people, cause nausea, diarrhoea and abdominal pain and should therefore be taken with care. Those who are elderly or who suffer weakness of the heart, liver or kidneys, or who have disorders of the digestive tract, should consider an alternative treatment.

Indomethacin is a powerful alternative to colchicine, though with similar side effects.

Allopurinol may be used to reduce levels of uric acid in the blood, even in those with kidney damage. It may actually cause attacks of gout in the early weeks of treatment, but seems to prevent attacks in the long term.

More information on these drugs is contained in chapter Two.

After an attack of gout, great care should be taken to avoid foods that create a lot of uric acid, such as offal. These foods contain high levels of purine, a substance which is converted into uric acid and then to urate crystals. Instead, fresh foods should be eaten and daily exercise taken to reduce the amount of uric acid in the blood. Drink plenty of water or clear fluid each day.

● Natural remedies: Diet (chapter 4), Supplements (chapter 4), Exercise (chapter 5), Lifestyle (chapter 6), Homoeopathy & Biochemics (chapter 7), Water (chapter 10), and From the East (chapter 11).

Infective Arthritis

● Osteomyelitis, Pott's disease, rheumatic fever and tuberculous arthritis are all forms of infective arthritis which are dealt with under separate headings.

● Bacteria can cause arthritis by invading a joint through the blood, lymph, joint fluid, or through infection already present in nearby tissues. Previous infection anywhere in the body, general ill-health or use of drugs which interfere with your defences can lower your resistance to infection, so early diagnosis and treatment of any puzzling symptoms is important.

The symptoms of an infective arthritis are similar to those of rheumatoid arthritis – starting with a general feeling of being unwell, fatigue, weight-loss, enlarged lymph glands and possible anaemia. There is sometimes fever and, of course, pain in one or two joints. A blood test or sample of the synovial fluid from a painful joint will reveal the bacterium causing the infection.

● Septic arthritis is caused by infection which is pyogenic, that is, it creates pus in the joint cavity. This can be very serious and rapid treatment must be given to prevent destruction of the joint and spread of the infection. Treatment consists of injections of an antibiotic as well as exercises to keep the joint from joining together (ankylosis). In rare cases, the joint must be opened up and drained of the accumulated pus.

● Gonococcal arthritis is a complication of the venereal disease gonorrhea and is caused by that bacterium. It is found most often in women because other initial symptoms of gonorrhea are not as obvious in women as in men, therefore early treatment of the disease is less likely. A single joint – e.g. the ankle, knee or wrist – is usually affected and it becomes hot, red and very painful. The soft tissue around the joint is also involved and may feel lumpy. Further symptoms include painful urination (in both men and women) and, in women, abdominal pain in the region of the ovaries. Vaginal discharge may occur.

● Diagnosis is confirmed by extracting some fluid from the afflicted joint and testing it for the infection. Treatment with antibiotics is generally effective.

● If any infection is left unattended it may destroy the joint completely and go on to attack the large organs of the body, causing severe and unnecessary damage. Early diagnosis usually means successful treatment. Infective arthritis should always be diagnosed and treated by your doctor. The recommended natural remedies should not be used *instead* of orthodox medical treatment, but may be used during and after medical treatment to speed your recovery.

● Natural remedies: Diet (chapter 4), Homoeopathy & Biochemics (chapter 7), and From the East (chapter 11).

Iritis SEE *Juvenile Rheumatoid Arthritis*

Juvenile Rheumatoid Arthritis
● Also called Still's disease, the first symptoms are a high fever, a rash on the middle body which comes and goes, and inflammation of the iris (the coloured part of the eye). This last symptom is called iritis and can appear weeks or months before the other signs of juvenile rheumatoid arthritis. In iritis, the iris and eyelid become swollen and painful, with some redness around the temple and blurred vision.

Swollen lymph glands usually accompany this disease and occasionally the spleen is enlarged. As in adult rheumatoid arthritis, one or more joints are afflicted with pain, swelling and limitation of movement.

● The juvenile form of rheumatoid arthritis occurs most commonly in children between 2 and 5 years of age. The child is usually clear of the disease by the time he or she reaches mid-teens.

The danger of deformity is greater in juvenile rheumatoid arthritis than in many adult cases because the child is growing. Therefore, it is essential that exercise and physiotherapy are maintained to keep the muscles strong and the joints mobile. Adequate rest – up to ten hours sleep each day – is essential to improve the child's general health.

● Drugs used in adult rheumatoid arthritis are sometimes used, with caution and under doctor's supervision, in the juvenile form. However, this is a very controversial subject. The Committee on Safety of Medicines has recently recommended that aspirin products should not be given to children under the age of twelve years except under strict control and in specially indicated cases of, for instance, juvenile rheumatoid arthritis. The effect of a drug on a child does not always coincide with its effect on an adult, hence the advisability of great caution.

● Natural remedies: Exercise (chapter 5), Water (chapter 10), and From the East (chapter 11).

Lumbago
● Also called lumbar rheumatism, this painful condition affects the area of spine at the small of your back around the five lumbar vertebrae (see diagram). Pain may be very sharp, acute and passing or dull, aching and chronic. Stiffness or total immobility of the area may affect you for a day or a week, depending on the severity and cause of the lumbago.

● There are at least a dozen possible causes of this disorder.

Among them are injury, stress, kidney infection, menstruation, obesity, loss of muscle tone, pregnancy, general illness such as cold or flu, and, of course, arthritis. Lumbago is a condition which many people will suffer from at least once in their lives. It is, in simple terms, a pain in the back! You should understand that lumbago may itself be a symptom of some other disorder and you must determine to resolve the primary problem if you wish to be rid of it.

● Pain relief and the reduction of any inflammation are the first steps in treating this disorder. After the pain has been eased, exercise or physiotherapy are necessary in order to keep your lumbar vertebrae mobile and the muscles of your back and abdomen strong and supple. This is especially important if you have a sedentary job, or frequently feel stressful. In both cases, exercise will improve your outlook, posture and the health of your lumbar spine.

THE SPINE AND PELVIS

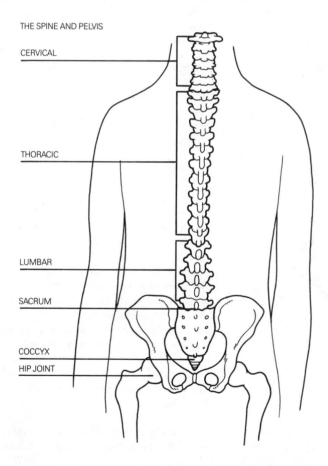

CERVICAL

THORACIC

LUMBAR

SACRUM

COCCYX

HIP JOINT

Pregnant women are also advised to exercise in order to maintain strength in their back throughout the changes in posture which are normal to pregnancy.

If you are overweight, it is very important to reduce as obesity complicates problems in the lower back. Finally, sleeping on a firm mattress and keeping the lumbar region of your back warm at all times will help to speed recovery.

● Natural remedies: Diet (chapter 4), Supplements (chapter 4), Exercise (chapter 5), Hands On and Lifestyle (chapter 6), Homoeopathy & Biochemics (chapter 7), Plants (chapter 8), Water (chapter 10), From the East (chapter 11).

Menopausal Arthritis

● Also called climactic arthritis and arthropathia ovaripriva, this disease affects some women during their menopause. Their knees, shoulders, elbows and some small joints become painful and inflamed.

● A deficiency of ovarian hormones is thought to be the cause of this arthritis, hence its appearance in women of menopausal age.

● If osteoporosis is also present, hormone replacement therapy (HRT) with oestrogens may be used to prevent this condition from worsening. In the short term, anti-inflammatory analgesics are used.

● Natural remedies: Diet (chapter 4), Exercise (chapter 5), Hands On and Lifestyle (chapter 6), Homoeopathy & Biochemics (chapter 7), Water (chapter 10), From the East (chapter 11).

Myositis

● Myositis is a rheumatic condition in which muscle becomes inflamed. There are many specific types of myositis, all of which bear the hallmark of inflammation which may sometimes extend to the skin. For instance, myositis fibrosa is inflammation of the muscle due to connective tissue growing within the muscle. In myositis ossificans bony tissue develops within the muscle and so causes inflammation, while myositis a frigore is inflammation of the muscle due simply to the cold. (See also Fibrositis.)

● Certain conditions predispose one to suffer from myositis. General poor health, poor living conditions and the cold may create opportunity for myositis to take hold and injury, infection or trauma may further contribute to the onset of this condition. Some forms of myositis are progressive and consequently your discomfort and disability increase. These cases are rare.

● Treatment must be given according to the precise nature of the disorder. General treatment involves warmth and the use of anti-inflammatory and pain-relieving drugs.

● Natural remedies: Exercise (chapter 5), Hands On and Lifestyle (chapter 6), Plants (chapter 8), Water (chapter 10), and From the East (chapter 11).

Neuritis
● This condition describes the inflammation of nerves anywhere in the body. It is a painful disorder which can result in a total or partial deadening of nerve sensation, muscle wastage and even paralysis. While not, strictly speaking, a rheumatic or arthritic disorder, neuritis can complicate or be mistaken for rheumatic or arthritic problems (see Sciatica).
● There are many causes of neuritis and some are affiliated with joint disorders. For instance, a nerve may become 'trapped' or compressed as a result of an arthritic condition which has altered a joint, or as a result of changes in joint alignment following injury or the delivery of a child. Other diseases, such as gout, can create metabolic changes which affect the health of your nerves. If nerve inflammation does eventually cause muscle wastage in a particular area of the body, that area may then become vulnerable to conditions which can cause arthritis.
● Treatment includes pain relief, rest and gentle exercise (in balanced amounts) to prevent loss of mobility. Heat applications and massage are soothing and help to maintain muscle tone and joint mobility. A diet high in vitamins and minerals will prevent further deterioration of general health.
● Natural remedies: Diet (chapter 4), Exercise (chapter 5), Hands On and Lifestyle (chapter 6), Homoeopathy & Biochemics (chapter 7), Water (chapter 10), and From the East (chapter 11).

Osteoarthritis
● This form of arthritis is non-inflammatory. It is also called degenerative joint disease and hypertrophic arthritis. The knees, hips, spine and small joints of the hands are most affected. Often the most rapid disease progress is in the weight-bearing regions of the body.

In osteoarthritis, the cartilage protecting the ends of bone in a joint degenerates, causing the bone edges to rub together. Damage is caused to the bone, which attempts to repair by over-producing bone tissue. The bony projections, called osteophytes, which result add to the overall degeneration of the joint and can cause further damage to the surrounding tissue. Pain and stiffness, especially after prolonged or strenuous activity, are the primary symptoms of osteoarthritis with pain very noticeable at night. Movement is limited and there can be muscle wastage and creaky joints (crepitis). This form of arthritis is famous for foretelling the weather.

NOTE: Crepitis is common in most people and does not, by itself, indicate osteoarthritis.

● Ageing is the primary cause of osteoarthritis – men and women over 55 years of age being equally vulnerable to it – but injury or dislocation of a joint can cause the symptoms at any age. This disease is often attributed to 'wear and tear' and in some cases this is so. For instance, obesity or excess weight placed continually on a joint – such as happens in one hip when the other is already weak or damaged – can cause osteoarthritis. Also, a continuous percussion in the joint can begin to cause changes which might later result in osteoarthritis; this is a concern held by people who are opposed to jogging as a form of exercise.

It is possible, however, that other factors ranging from diet to stress may precipitate the onset of osteoarthritis. The fact that menopausal women are also vulnerable to it indicates that metabolic changes are, at least in part, responsible for some cases of osteoarthritis.

● Pain relief is an important treatment in this disease. Both rest and exercise are also necessary, although the exercise must be gentle and taken regularly. If adequate rest cannot be achieved at night, then naps must be taken during the day to make up for lost sleep. If you are overweight, it is important to reduce as this will relieve the pressure on any weight-bearing joints which suffer. Some people find that a walking stick or frame is helpful if their hips and legs are involved.

Surgical treatment of osteoarthritis has advanced rapidly of late; the most successful operation is probably the 'hip replacement'. There are two forms. In arthroplasty, an acrylic head is attached to the thigh bone within the hip joint. This, on recovery, allows movement at the hip. Arthrodesis, the second method, fixes the hip joint with a metal plate and pin so that movement is not possible. Growth of bone over this pin is encouraged by implanting chips of bone. This is sometimes called artificial ankylosis. Both operations usually result in freedom from pain after a period of recovery.

Osteoarthritis is a degenerative disease and therefore gets worse. However, pain relief, rest, weight loss and gentle exercise can prevent it progressing too rapidly. Deformity is not a part of this condition.

● Natural remedies: Diet (chapter 4), Exercise (chapter 5), Hands On and Lifestyle (chapter 6), Remedies That You Wear (chapter 9), Water (chapter 10), From the East (chapter 11).

Osteomyelitis

● In osteomyelitis the bone and bone marrow become inflamed through infection. A very strong, deep pain is an early symptom, accompanied by a high fever and sweating. The muscles around the affected bone are swollen, very tender and the presence of pus may be obvious. If the pus enters a joint cavity it can cause gross destruction to it.

● Infection in other areas of the body, for instance the lungs, can be passed through the bloodstream to cause osteomyelitis. This process is more likely in children and is most often caused by the staphylococcus bacterium.

In adults, the more usual cause is injury to the bone, such as a fracture or 'chipping'. A piece of bone which has actually separated from its parent bone will die and become a source of infection itself. The appearance of this disease in the spine is partly due to damaged vertebrae and partly to reduced blood flow to the vertebral joints. In fact, the likelihood of bone infection occurring through injury is greatly enhanced if you also suffer from an arterial disease.

● Treatment must be immediate. An antibiotic is generally given in large doses so that the infection is killed and not simply disguised. The pus from infection is drawn out through a needle or the area is opened surgically and the infection drained. If a bone chip (sequestrum) is present, an operation is necessary in order to remove it. In all cases, some degree of immobility must be imposed on the area until the infection has cleared. Osteomyelitis should always be diagnosed and treated by your doctor. The recommended natural remedies should not be used instead of orthodox medical treatment, but may be used during and after medical treatment to speed your recovery.

● Natural remedies: Supplements (chapter 4) and Homoeopathy & Biochemics (chapter 7).

Osteoporosis

● In this disease the bones lose their strength and density, becoming brittle and easy to break. The hips and spine are most affected, possibly because they take your body's weight. General back pain, occasionally centred in the lower back, rounding shoulders, some height loss and easy fractures occur later in the development of osteoporosis. Osteoporosis gives few indications in its early stages.

● Post-menopausal women are most susceptible to this disease and of those, fair-skinned women who are also thin are particularly vulnerable. This is due to their lower level of oestrogen production and the subsequent lower level of circulating oestrogen. Adequate levels of circulating oestrogen are needed for your body to retain the calcium taken in your diet and osteoporosis is thought to be caused, in part, by insufficient calcium retained in the body.

● Diet in early life is believed to determine, to some extent, the likelihood of suffering from osteoporosis in later life. In particular, the quantities of calcium and vitamin D present in your early diet (infancy to adolescence) determine the strength and density of bone throughout our lives. A calcium-rich diet in the childbearing years (20–40) will help to maintain bone density, which could otherwise be lost in the development of a child. By the menopause, your body's ability to absorb calcium is reduced and so more attention must be given to ensuring a calcium-rich diet. Supplementation of the diet in later years is beneficial but not entirely preventative. A combination of vitamins and minerals makes up a worthwhile supplementation, with vitamin D, calcium, protein and possibly oestrogen included. It is worth noting that smoking reduces the level of circulating oestrogen and may therefore aggravate this condition.

Analgesics are often given to relieve pain, but this is really only valid if consistent, gentle exercise is also taken to maintain or improve mobility. Exercise stimulates your metabolism, in particular your body's ability to use the calcium present in your diet. Osteoporosis can actually be aggravated by lack of exercise, because all of your metabolic processes become sluggish or function incorrectly. Walking is one of the best forms of exercise.

Osteoporosis is a progressive disease, though for some its presence is not crippling. Attitude and activity are important aspects of any treatment.

● Natural remedies: Diet (chapter 4), Supplements (chapter 4), Exercise (chapter 5) and Homoeopathy & Biochemics (chapter 7).

Paget's Disease
● Also called osteitis deformans, this disease consists of simultaneous bone rarefaction (loss of density) and excessive bone growth. The result is a patchiness in the density of the bones which makes them weak and liable to fracture, as in osteoporosis, while the new, excessive bone growth often causes deformity. This disease takes years, or even decades, to develop and therefore the symptoms do not appear until late in life, if at all.

Symptoms are vague, deep pains in the bones which shift around the body with possible deforming of the legs, spine, pelvis and skull. In particular, the legs may bow, the spine may curve or lose height and the skull may become enlarged. Changes in the skull will probably cause headaches and loss of hearing. Spontaneous fractures or other problems requiring X-ray, may lead to the diagnosis of Paget's disease.

● Symptoms usually appear in people over 50 years of age with twice as many men as women suffering but because the development of Paget's disease is so gradual, the actual onset may occur any time after the age of 30 years. The cause of this condition is unknown.

● X-ray may tell the extent of the disease but no remedy is known. Mild pain relief may be given over a long period of time with occasional use of radiotherapy to reduce discomfort. However, the best outlook is to keep moving to avoid becoming an invalid.

● Natural remedies: Exercise (chapter 5) and Hands On and Lifestyle (chapter 6).

Palindromic Rheumatism

● In this disorder there is inflammation of the tissues around a joint which comes and goes repeatedly. However, no permanent changes occur in the joints or in the surrounding tissue. Symptoms are the same as for arthritis with pain, stiffness and loss of mobility while the attack lasts. There is no fever.

● There is little known as to the cause of palindromic rheumatism. A number of factors may have a bearing on the start of an attack, such as weather, diet, emotional upset, fatigue, or general stress.

● Treatment should focus on basic health care. Get plenty of rest, improve your diet, keep warm and keep a very positive attitude so that you don't think yourself into feeling worse. Fortunately, this disease does not cause permanent damage.

● Natural remedies: Diet (chapter 4), Exercise (chapter 5), Hands On and Lifestyle (chapter 6), Plants (chapter 8) and From the East (chapter 11).

Poncet's Rheumatism

● That is also called tuberculous arthritis or tuberculous rheumatism. A high temperature and sweating at night is an early symptom of this disorder and may be accompanied by pain and weakness. Usually only one joint is affected but as movement is restricted early in the disease, rather than in the late stages, treatment should be sought immediately. The knees, hips and spine are usually at risk (for tuberculosis affecting specifically the spine see Pott's disease) and deformity or handicap can result if the disease is left untreated.

● Poncet's rheumatism is caused by the tubercle baccillus, the same bacterium which causes tuberculosis of the lungs. When a bone becomes infected, an abscess forms which destroys the bone tissue and eventually spreads to the joint. The disease continues to work there, creating pain, swelling and muscle spasm in the process. Even when the pain diminishes and the swelling subsides, the tuberculosis is still active. Symptoms will repeatedly flare up and then disappear.

Children are generally considered most vulnerable, although the incidence of tuberculosis has been greatly reduced in this country through the pasteurization of milk, the elimination of bovine tuberculosis and wide-spread vaccination.

● Early treatment is as for tuberculosis of the lungs and includes antibiotic and anti-tuberculous drug treatment. If necessary, a joint may be opened through surgery and the abscess removed. Occasionally, in a very advanced stage of disease, artificial ankylosis is created to prevent paralysis. Poncet's rheumatism is rarely seen and must always receive medical diagnosis and treatment.

● Natural remedies: Diet (chapter 4) and Water (chapter 10).

Pott's Disease

● This is tuberculosis of the spine, also called David's disease, dorsal phthisis and spondylitis tuberculosa. It can affect the vertebrae themselves or the connective tissue which surrounds them and results in inflammation and eventual enlargement of the vertebrae. High fever with night sweats, some abdominal pain as well as pain in the spine are early symptoms. There is difficulty in moving and a gradual curvature of the spine can result, eventually forming a humpback.

● The cause of Pott's disease is the tubercle baccillus. Fortunately it is now a rare disease due to the eradication of bovine tuberculosis, widespread vaccination and the pasteurization of milk.

● Rest and improved general health are important beginnings of any treatment. If diagnosed early, antibiotic and anti-tuberculous drugs are used as treatment. In some cases a splint or brace is used to support the spine while the drug treatment is in progress. This is to prevent deformity and promote healing by eliminating pressure and friction. Untreated cases can result in deformity and paralysis. Pott's disease must always receive medical diagnosis and treatment.

● Natural remedies: Diet (chapter 4) and Water (chapter 10).

Psychogenic Rheumatism

● This form of rheumatism has an emotional or psychological beginning. It may be used to describe many of the more specific forms of rheumatic diseases if their cause is thought to stem from your mental or emotional state.

A psychogenic disease is one which may have begun after a time of great trauma, anxiety, grief or other mental or emotional stress. These states alter your physical health by affecting all of your basic body functions. There is nothing abnormal in this, but in some people these changes trigger off a disease process.

● Treatment will vary according to the type of disease which manifests. Your doctor may recommend anything from antidepressants to counselling sessions or yoga classes.

● Natural remedies: Exercise (chapter 5), Hands On (chapter 6), Plants (chapter 8), From the East (chapter 11).

Rheumatic Fever

● This is a dangerous childhood disease which induces, as just one part of its activity, acute rheumatoid arthritis. Rheumatic fever usually follows an infection of the throat, caused normally by the streptococcus bacterium. It begins with a high fever and attacks of arthritis in the large joints. The arthritis then moves on to the smaller joints, and the attacks continue to move around the body in this manner. The joints become very painful, swollen, red and hot. Sometimes nodules appear around the joints and this is often an indication that the heart is involved. Apart from the sweating and loss of appetite associated with the fever, there is usually a rapid pulse. This is an important symptom because rheumatic fever can also cause inflammation of the heart. The valves of the heart may become deformed as a result and heart problems may be encountered later in life. The most feared effect of rheumatic fever is Chorea which is inflammation of the brain tissue.

● Children are most vulnerable between the ages of 7 and 12 years. It was thought that cold, damp and poverty were the cause of the fever. But it now seems that overcrowding – no matter how poor or wealthy the family – contributes most to this disease being contracted.

● Bed rest and antibiotics are the best and most immediate treatment. Bed rest may be necessary for several weeks. The antibiotics act to clear the disease from the body and so are preferable to aspirin and the cortisone group, which relieve pain but are not curative, simply masking the symptoms.

Once out of the sick-bed, a victim of rheumatic fever must have a strong blend of rest and activity, with a good diet and a positive attitude. Full recovery takes several months.

● Rheumatic fever requires medical diagnosis and treatment.

Rheumatoid Arthritis
● Also called arthritis deformans, proliferative arthritis and rheumatic gout, rheumatoid arthritis is often abbreviated to simply RA. It is both inflammatory and degenerative and can affect any and all of the body's joints, from toes to jaw. Early symptoms are general – brief pains in the small joints along with fatigue and morning stiffness – and may precede the full-blown attack of RA by several weeks. However, as the disease takes hold, the pain will persist, sometimes becoming quite piercing. At the same time, swelling of the tissues around the painful joints occurs, including the ligaments and tendons. This inflammation gradually affects both the synovial membrane and the cartilage and thus begins the destruction of the joint.

The additional degeneration of the fibrous connective tissues surrounding a joint can cause the muscles to become wasted. This process in turn speeds the destruction of the joint, resulting ultimately in ankylosis (the joint growing together). Certainly, in this disease the joints affected tend to deform.

There is little rhyme or reason in the way rheumatoid arthritis manifests in the body. For instance, it can present itself in one or two small joints and remain there, unchanged, for a considerable time. Then suddenly it will progress to include several more joints all at once. Also, the intensity of the pain will vary from day to day and great suffering can alternate with times of relative freedom from discomfort.

● Two to three times as many women as men suffer from rheumatoid arthritis and most sufferers are in their 30s or 40s. No one knows the cause of RA. It seems likely that stress, especially sudden and severe stress, can bring on the symptoms and that this tendency may also 'run in the family'. (Perhaps because family members learn similar ways of dealing with stress?) Some suggestions have been made that RA is in some way a reaction of the body against itself – as though it had become confused. If this is so, it is called an auto-immune disease.

● Rheumatoid arthritis cannot be cured. That is the bad news. The good news is that it can be pushed into a corner of your life instead of taking it over. Treatment takes two forms: attendance to general health and the use of anti-inflammatory and pain relief substances.

General health may be improved by getting plenty of rest, eating a very nutritious diet and keeping mobile. Rest may be improved by using a duvet instead of blankets to keep pressure off the joints. Diet should be iron-rich to counteract the tendency to anaemia, and gentle exercise should become a part of your daily life.

Aspirin is a popular treatment for inflammation and pain; however, it is unsuitable for long-term, frequent use. Other treatments include non-steroidal anti-inflammatory drugs, gold salts, anti-malarial drugs, steroids and ACTH hormone therapies. Please look under their separate headings for detailed information about their effect.

Occasionally, the use of splints and braces is advised. These may be useful in the short term to relieve pain and swelling. In the long term, they encourage wastage of the muscles and should therefore not be considered a remedy.

● Natural remedies: Diet (chapter 4), Supplements (chapter 4), Exercise (chapter 5), Hands On and Lifestyle (chapter 6), Remedies that You Wear (chapter 9), Water (chapter 10) and From the East (chapter 11).

Sciatica

● The sciatic nerve runs from the lumbar region of the spine (see diagram on page 17) right down the legs and into the feet. Irritation of this nerve results in sciatica – a severe and overwhelming pain in the buttocks and down the back of one leg. The pain is sometimes described as 'shooting', although usually a background ache is present all of the time.

● Sciatica is usually caused by pressure against the sciatic nerve near where it joins the spine or where it passes through the pelvis into the leg. Pressure can be caused by inflamed organs or blood vessels, or by changes in pelvic or vertebral joints due to arthritis or injury. Anyone can suffer from sciatica, although general good health makes the condition less likely. Poor posture, sitting still for a long period of time or an unaccustomed burst of activity can all combine to bring on sciatica. Cold and damp will make it worse.

● The best treatment is prevention. Strong muscles in your back, abdomen and buttocks as well as good posture both sitting and standing are important means of prevention. Correct use of your back while lifting, carrying or pushing an object are also important skills to acquire.

Resting on a firm mattress or the floor with heat applied to the lower back will provide initial treatment during an attack of sciatica. Aspirin may be useful to relieve pain and any accompanying inflammation. But after initial relief is obtained, the cause of the irritation must be resolved. This may mean dealing with a 'slipped' disc or other vertebral problems, undertaking physiotherapy or an exercise regime for the back and legs, or simply having a massage.

The pain of sciatica is debilitating and attention should be given to diet and rest. The problem will recur unless corrective steps are taken, in particular those which will strengthen the body and improve your posture and ways of moving.

● Natural remedies: Exercise (chapter 5), Hands On and Lifestyle (chapter 6), Homoeopathy & Biochemics (chapter 7), Water (chapter 10) and From the East (chapter 11).

Spondylitis

● Spondylitis is a general term for inflammation of the vertebrae and may be of several types. Its early symptoms are pain and stiffness in the pelvis and lumbar region of the spine – sometimes called lumbago (see separate heading). Inflammation is not apparent and the disorder gradually progresses up the spine to include the ribs and neck. In its later stages it is ankylosing spondylitis (see separate heading) because the inflammation damages the joints and they begin to fuse together.

● Young men are most vulnerable to this disorder. It is considered a rheumatic complaint but the cause of spondylitis is unknown, although an injury, illness or persistent misuse of the back may encourage the development of the first symptoms.

● Correct posture at all times, including sleeping on a firm mattress, eases the discomfort and prevents curvature of the spine. Pain relief includes non-steroidal anti-inflammatory drugs and the range of drugs used for rheumatoid arthritis. Occasionally, radiotherapy is used during hospital treatment especially in the later stages when the ribs may be included. There is risk of leukaemia with over-use of radiotherapy treatment. Surgery, splints and braces are sometimes employed to prevent deformity.

● Natural remedies: Hands On and Lifestyle (chapter 6), Water (chapter 10) and From the East (chapter 11).

Still's Disease SEE Juvenile Rheumatoid Arthritis

Synovitis

● This is a general term used to describe inflammation of the synovial membrane. Such inflammation occurs in most forms of arthritis and it always causes pain on movement and periods of apparent swelling. Synovitis involving the bursae is often called bursitis, while that involving a tendon sheath is often called tenosynovitis (see separate headings).

● Synovitis can occur in any joint (or bursa or tendon). This painful disorder may be caused by infection, injury, over-use of the afflicted joint, or as a companion to another rheumatic disease. Anyone may suffer from it.

● Treatment includes heat, poultices and liniment rubs, rest, and non-steroidal anti-inflammatory drugs.
● Natural remedies: Hands On and Lifestyle (chapter 6), Water (chapter 10) and From the East (chapter 11).

Tendinitis
● This disorder is commonly suffered in the shoulder and ankle areas. It is an inflammation of the tendon or of the tendon and nearby muscle. It is sometimes called calcific bursitis due to the thickening of the tendon and the calcification of nearby bursae (see also Bursitis).
● The cause of tendinitis seems to be over-use, or sudden and extreme challenges to the tendon such as a new sport or a very long walk on hard pavement.
● Rest is the first treatment used, in an attempt to reduce the inflammation. Ultra-sound has been of value in breaking down calcific deposits, combined with physiotherapy to regain mobility. Application of heat helps to relieve the tenderness on moving, and aspirin or other non-steroidal anti-inflammatory drugs may provide some additional pain relief. Surgery is occasionally employed to remove calcific deposits.
● Natural remedies: Supplements (chapter 4), Hands On and Lifestyle (chapter 6) and From the East (chapter 11).

Tenosynovitis
● This is the name given to an inflammation of the synovial sheath surrounding a tendon. There are two forms, simple and suppurative (producing pus). Both cause distress, although the suppurative form restricts movement much more than the simple form.
● Infection, as from gonorrhea or tuberculosis, can invade the tendon sheath and surrounding tissue and cause inflammation. Over-use or a sharp injury may also result in inflammation of the tendon sheath.
● Rest, pain relief and massage aid the simple form of tenosynovitis, while penicillin and sulphonomides are needed to remedy the suppurative form. Sometimes the suppuration must be drained, requiring an incision.
● Natural remedies: Hands On and Lifestyle (chapter 6) and From the East (chapter 11).

Tuberculous Arthritis
● Tuberculosis is an inflammatory disease caused by infection from the tubercle baccillus. Generally, the bacterium is inhaled or swallowed and from there spreads through the blood to the organs and tissues of the body.
● See Poncet's disease and Pott's disease for the specific effects of tuberculosis on the bones and joints.

Prevention, Relief and Cure: How much is Possible?

It very much depends on the problem! Bursitis, for instance, can enjoy all three: prevent it by buying shoes that fit or sharing your work between both arms, relieve it with any number of natural or orthodox treatments, and cure it with time, treatment and yet another dose of prevention.

Prevention is the best cure. You may know things now which could help others prevent a rheumatic disorder in themselves, even if you are too late to prevent it in yourself. Yet, you may be able to prevent your own problem getting worse or any more complicated by doing your utmost to gain and retain health.

Relief is easily obtained from many sources and you may even find yourself spoiled for choice. But of course, you should simply use the form of relief which best suits you: your disorder, your needs and your long-term health goals. You can create your own health programme from the variety of orthodox and natural treatments which follow.

Cure is elusive, except in those cases obviously temporary and the result of, say, injury. But this term needs to be put into perspective. Many people improve the quality of their lives to the extent that they rarely think of their disorder, although clinically they are still afflicted.

All medicine, orthodox and natural, strives to accomplish cure. Both strive equally to prevent disease. But relief remains the common ground, the state in which most sufferers live, with their symptoms more or less prominent.

Your ultimate state of health or disease does not lie solely with the medicines you use, however, it lies with you. Your attitude and your level of determination decide, in the final count, how much health is really possible for you.

2

The Causes
of
Rheumatism
and Arthritis

The cause of rheumatic disease is still difficult to pin down. Specific diseases have their specific symptoms and treatments and contributory factors, and some of the disease processes are well understood, well tested and well observed. Yet the actual cause of many of the rheumatic diseases is still described as 'suspected'.

The rheumatic diseases seem to be holistic diseases – that is, they tend to involve the whole of your body as well as your mental and emotional state, however much the symptoms and discomforts are centred in one area or joint. Perhaps finding the cause of rheumatic disease is so elusive because the cause is many-faceted!

In this section some of the major factors contributing to the rheumatic diseases are discussed. Most diseases could easily seem to have more than one of these factors as their starting point. In your first visit to your GP, you may wish to mention what you think started your problem. In many cases, your opinion will be as important as one of the diagnostic tests.

Ageing and Change of Life

The rheumatic diseases can strike at any time but certain forms of them are specific to ageing or the change of life in women. The risk of suffering from rheumatism or arthritis usually has more to do with previous injury, ill health and various nutritional deficiencies than it does with simply getting older. It's just that sometimes these problems don't become obvious for several years by which time you may be – well – old! Ageing causes a gradual change in the structure and processes of every cell in your body and these changes can encourage some forms of rheumatism or arthritis to develop from early misfortune.

The changes and reduction in hormone production as a woman goes through the menopause, or change of life, have effect on her general health. For some women, these changes exacerbate rheumatic or arthritic conditions, including demineralization – a loss of essential minerals. A well-known result of demineralization is osteoporosis.

Diet and Deficiency Related Causes

There is an on-going controversy as to whether poor diet and deficiency in vitamins and minerals actually causes rheumatic or arthritic conditions. The discussion divides into three parts. The first denies that diet influences the disease at all. The second looks at the person already suffering and attempts to remedy their problem by improving their diet or supplementing it with vitamins and minerals. The third viewpoint sees diet, vitamins and minerals as important in preventing disorders. In particular, this third viewpoint is concerned with infancy, childhood and even the diet of parents affecting their unborn children. The contention is that good health established early on in life supports good health in later life. This theory is currently under study to gain scientific validity, but many people feel that it is common sense to suppose that the theory is correct.

Many of us, entering our middle and late decades, are possibly living the effects of our early diet with all of its excesses and deficiencies. If any of these early patterns do, in fact, contribute to the development of rheumatism and arthritis then you must do your utmost to prevent similar dietary patterns being established in the young people you know. You might also do your best to correct the deficiencies and excesses in your current daily life by changing or supplementing your diet. Who knows? You may reduce your suffering in the process.

Emotional and Environmental Causes

Emotion is partly dependent on the levels of certain hormones in your body. So when an emotional trauma or a period of difficulty in your emotional life occurs, your hormones change to deal with the stress of this time. Certain hormonal changes can bring about attacks of arthritis or rheumatism because of the effects these changes have on the way your body functions. While *you* may feel queasy or nervous or depressed, your muscles, joints and connective tissues may suffer other side effects of hormonal change – namely, arthritis or rheumatism. Rheumatoid arthritis is the most severe rheumatic disorder which can be brought about by emotional causes and other, possibly more transient, conditions such as lumbago, fibrositis, ganglion and 'frozen shoulder' may also derive from emotional problems.

Environmental causes of rheumatism and arthritis are very much under the 'suspected' heading. For instance, it is widely felt, but not proven, that rheumatic fever is more prevalent in over-crowded conditions, as already mentioned. And cold damp climates or housing conditions pave the way for many rheumatic and arthritic complaints.

Hereditary and Genetic Causes

Errors in metabolism can be passed on within a family. The rheumatic diseases attributed, at least in part, to inherited traits are gout and osteoporosis. Both rheumatoid arthritis and ankylosing spondylitis are suspected of being inherited tendencies. Inherited weaknesses of the circulation and digestion may create opportunities for a rheumatic disease to establish.

Infection

This is the cause of many rheumatic and arthritic conditions. Infection is most often caused by the tubercle baccillus or the staphylococcal, streptococcal or gonococcal bacteria. These infections usually initiate at the site of a wound, in the lungs or through venereal contact and are spread throughout your body by the blood or lymph.

When infection establishes in or near a joint, a process of destruction begins which includes the synovial membrane, connective tissues, cartilage and eventually the bone itself. The joint may become filled with fluid or pus, ulcers may develop and inflammation will occur. Infection of any sort draws on your body's resources to deal with it. Anaemia usually results from prolonged inflammation and this further depletes your body's fighting capabilities.

Injury, Inactivity and Wear and Tear

A sharp blow to a bone or joint, a fracture, a dislocation, even surgery – all these types of injury may contribute to the development of a rheumatic or arthritic condition. Any of these injuries may allow infection into the joint or surrounding tissue, creating an opportunity for the infection to do its work. Or the injury may cause immediate damage to the joint or surrounding tissue so that factors such as cold and damp, de-mineralization, or wear and tear increase the damage and speed destruction of the joint.

'Wear and tear' may be thought of as gradual injury. Over a period of time – sometimes decades – the natural ageing process, obesity, or over-exertion of some sort creates stress and minor injury to the joint which can later promote rheumatic and arthritic disorders. Injury and wear and tear can occur at any point in your life and still have a bearing on later health. Discussion continues, for instance, concerning the jogging and aerobics fashions and their wear and tear effect on the feet, ankles, knees, hips and lower spine. Obesity is thought to be hard on the knees, hips and lower back and obese arthritis sufferers are usually advised to reduce their weight to make treatment more effective. Many sufferers are not obese but are, in fact, under-weight, due partly to the debilitating effect of pain.

Before you become overly concerned about any invisible injury you may be causing yourself, please remember that *inactivity* can also contribute to some rheumatic disorders – such as osteoporosis. Your body is designed to move and if you don't keep it moving, you become prone to injury. Your muscles lose their tone, your bones lose density and your metabolism becomes sluggish. This is one 'cause' over which you have a great deal of control.

Other Illnesses or Medications

As described in the section on Infection, other illnesses are sometimes liable to act as a catalyst, or predispose you, to a rheumatic disorder. Any illness reduces your body's strength and stamina and this low resistance and general poor health can cause disturbances in your immune system which enable a rheumatic disorder to develop unrestricted.

Illness which is caused by taking medicine for another illness is called 'iatrogenic illness'. It is essentially a drug side effect, except the emphasis is usually long term. Some drugs can aggravate a rheumatic disorder, others can leave your body in a poor condition − susceptible to infection, for instance − and thus invite additional health problems.

All of the drugs used to treat the rheumatic diseases have side effects which may create additional problems for you. For instance, nausea, vertigo and skin rash might result just from taking aspirin. Iatrogenic illness is a real issue and before you begin any drug treatment you should discuss its possible long- and short-term side effects with your doctor.

How the Doctor makes a Diagnosis

There is a point of view among some doctors that diagnosis is never complete until the patient is well. This is quite true − you are always changing, and what feels like imminent demise one day may feel like a small niggle the next. A medical diagnosis must take all of your basic health features into account − including the quality of being human and therefore changeable.

There are several steps in making a diagnosis and your doctor will use them in the order which he or she finds works best. A diagnosis is essential if your condition is to be treated early and effectively, but your GP needs your help to make a correct diagnosis. If you understand the information he or she requires, and are able to give it, then a lot of time and probably suffering will be saved. When you talk with your doctor be as accurate, precise and thorough as you can.

Your Family Medical History

If your doctor knows you or has received your old medical notes, this section will not apply to your visit. However, if this is your first visit to your GP, he or she may take your medical history (this will include some information about your family's medical background, too). Your doctor will probably note your history beginning with your childhood. For instance:

Q   What diseases have you suffered from in the past?
Q   Did any of these affect your muscles or joints?
Q   Did you have, for instance, rheumatic fever? Chorea? Juvenile rheumatoid arthritis?

Q   Has any member of your family suffered from gout, rheumatoid arthritis, ankylosing spondylitis, or other forms of arthritis?

Q   Is there a history of diabetes, hypertension, or heart disease in your family?

History-taking requires a bit of time, which is why more time is usually allotted you on your first visit to a GP. Once it is done, each subsequent visit can begin in the present. Your doctor will want to know how you are in general before getting on to the specifics of your complaint. If you know your doctor well, he or she can probably tell a lot about how you are feeling just by the way you enter the room and sit down. In any case, your doctor should ask you a few questions about your general well-being, such as:

Q   Are you happy in your work?

Q   Are you happy in your home life?

Q   Are you using any medication for any reason at the present?

Q   How much sleep do you get, on average, each night?

He or she will also observe your general appearance, such as posture, colouring, balance and ease in movement before beginning to note the symptoms of your complaint.

Noting Your Symptoms: Main and Secondary

You must talk a lot, even if you are unsure your doctor wants to hear it. The information you provide is necessary and if you hold back you may make it difficult for your doctor to make a correct diagnosis. Without the diagnosis, the doctor may be unable to provide appropriate treatment.

Main symptoms: When you describe your symptoms you should aim to recreate them in your doctor's mind, so be precise about the timing and intensity of your symptoms without, of course, exaggerating. Your doctor will ask questions to help you supply the information needed.

● Describe WHAT you are feeling, i.e. pain, ache, throbbing, stabbing.

● Describe WHERE you are feeling it, i.e. wrists, knees, back, neck.

● Describe WHEN you feel it MOST and LEAST, i.e. most at night, least after walking back from the shops.

● Tell WHEN your symptoms began. Include dates and times of day if you can remember them.

● Tell HOW LONG the first occurrence lasted.

● Tell HOW it affected your work, sleep and daily activities.

● Tell whether the symptoms MOVED to other areas of your body.

In addition, your doctor will want to know whether you have treated your symptoms yourself and, if so, the details of the treatment. Some treatments have side-effects which may confuse your original symptoms, so your doctor must know what you have taken so that he or she may focus on the original problem. Therefore,

● Tell WHAT TREATMENT you have taken, if any
● Describe the DOSE, FREQUENCY and DURATION of the treatment
● Describe any side effects you think you may have had, if any.

Secondary symptoms: Usually pain, swelling and difficulty in moving are considered 'main' symptoms – if only because they are so definite and intrude into your life. Secondary symptoms are more the sort of symptoms you can live with; they are discomforts which lie more in the background of your life, but they are still important to reveal. Your doctor might ask you questions which may seem, at first, irrelevant to your discomfort. For example:

Q   What time do you get up in the morning?
Q   Do you feel that your joints are stiff when you first get up?
Q   What time do you stop feeling stiff and begin to feel 'loosened up'?
Q   Do you feel tired at any particular point in the day? For instance, almost immediately you get up, mid-afternoon, early evening?
Q   Do any of your limbs or your movements feel weak to you?
Q   Do you have other complaints such as headache, constipation, skin problems or night sweats?

From information such as this, your doctor will begin putting together a picture of your disorder. More information can be gained from the following procedures, when you probably won't need to talk.

Physical Examination
Your doctor will usually remain silent, except to ask you to change position. You may be asked to remove some or all of your clothing. A physical examination includes:

Palpation: The doctor applies pressure to various joints of your body without wishing to cause pain, but hoping to sense any tenderness. The purpose is to learn if there is inflammation (apparent or non-apparent) and, if so, how much.

Range of motion: The doctor will ask you to get into a specific position and will then move, for instance, your arm or lower leg or wrist for you. In some cases, you will be asked to do a movement by yourself while the doctor applies pressure to the area around that joint. The object is to see how much your movement has been impaired, if at all. During the movement, the doctor will feel for any slight creaking (called crepitis) of the joints. Most people creak a certain amount and your doctor will be feeling to determine if the creaking is part of your problem, or just the air pockets and sliding tendons that are often the cause of crepitis.

Pressure (palpation) is applied again in order to learn how much muscle or connective tissue is involved in your problem, if any. Your doctor may advise you to perform one or two movements daily, at home, to maintain mobility in the affected joint or area of your body.

Observation: Your posture, general manner of moving and any swelling, lumpiness or bony growths will be noted. The doctor may touch the larger joints, such as the hips, to sense any heat and you may be asked to grip your doctor's wrist or finger to test for any weakness.

Following the physical examination, and depending on the pattern of symptoms your doctor has observed so far, you may be asked to undergo a test or series of tests. Tests are by no means fail safe and your doctor will usually use a test only to confirm the diagnosis he or she suspects. Don't feel that a test is necessary in order to complete a diagnosis – it isn't.

Blood Tests

The **erythrocyte sedimentation rate** test measures the speed that red blood cells settle to the bottom of a vertical tube in the course of one hour. If they settle quickly, in other words if a lot settle within that time, then it indicates that there is disease, inflammation or infection. If the red blood cells settle more slowly, then health is good or improving. Your doctor may already suspect you have, for instance, an infection and this test will confirm or disprove those suspicions *without indicating which infection is present*. If an infection is present, this test may be used regularly to learn when the infection becomes inactive. Similarly, if other disease or inflammatory conditions are suspected, their activity can be monitored by the ESR without the disease specifications.

● Certain proteins exist in your blood which have antibiotic characteristics. They are called immunoglobulins. A special variety of immunoglobulin – called the rheumatoid factor – exists in the blood of a person suffering from rheumatoid arthritis and a **blood serum test** will reveal this. However, people without RA may also have the rheumatoid factor, as may healthy people or those with other diseases. The ratio of the rheumatoid factor in the blood must therefore be quite high in order to support a tentative diagnosis of rheumatoid arthritis.

● Two further tests are often used and these are the **white blood cell count** and the **haematocrit** or red blood cell count. The white blood cell count is high when you are fighting an infection or suffering from the side effects of a drug so this test can tell the doctor whether, for instance, you are winning the fight or if you need to stop using a particular drug.

The red blood cell count, haematocrit, is low if, for instance, you are bleeding internally or if a drug you are taking causes decreased production of the red blood cells. Inflammation, especially if it is suffered over a long period of time, can also cause a drop in the red blood cell count so this test may be performed regularly if you have a rheumatic disorder.

Temperature, Pulse and Blood Pressure

These tests are fairly standard and certainly painless. They help your doctor to know more about your general health and whether another illness or chronic condition may be contributing to your problem.

● A rise in your body temperature is an indication that your body is fighting an infection. It is a natural reaction, or defence, against invading bacteria.

● Pulse is measured by rate, which is increased in some illnesses, by volume, such as a 'pounding' pulse during fever, and by rhythm, which may be regular or irregular.

● Blood pressure is raised – hypertension – with kidney disorders or with circulatory problems. Your doctor considers raised blood pressure an important factor in both diagnosis and prescribing treatment for you as some drugs should not be used in the case of hypertension.

Urine Sample

If gout is suspected, your doctor may test specifically for excess uric acid but generally a urine test will also determine if red blood cells, protein or urinary casts are present. Urinary casts are proteins or bacteria which mould together in the kidneys and are then passed out in the urine. Normal urine does not contain protein or casts and very few red blood cells. A test which shows up one of these substances will help your doctor judge the precise nature and progress of your disorder.

X-ray

An X-ray shows bony tissue clearly and therefore it can reveal destruction of a joint, the presence of bony growths and, of course, fractures and dislocations. It does not show problems with the soft tissues nearly so clearly and this means that an X-ray is not an essential part of the tests you will undergo. There is a danger associated with exposure to X-rays, which is radiation, and so it is wise to avoid them unless your doctor thinks an X-ray will provide necessary information or therapy.

Joint Fluid Tests

For this test a needle is inserted into the painful joint and some of the joint fluid removed. A number of tests may then be performed on this fluid, but the two most revealing of them test for infection or for sodium urate crystals. If infection is found, it can be named and the necessary treatment given; if urate crystals are present, a gouty arthritis is diagnosed and the specific treatment for that disease may be given.

It is possible that the tests necessary for a diagnosis of your complaint will not be performed all at once, if at all, so you may visit your GP but not know of a confirmed diagnosis till some time later. In this event, it is likely that your doctor will advise you regarding pain relief, posture, diet and ways of moving which will ease your discomfort until the diagnosis is complete.

Once the diagnosis is made ask your doctor to give you the name of the disorder and the details of it. If necessary, write the name of the condition down on a slip of paper so that you can learn more about it in your own time. Listen carefully to what is said and ask questions if you don't understand any part of the explanation. Following a diagnosis, the doctor will probably recommend a treatment.

Treatments Your Doctor May Suggest

It is useful to understand the purpose of the more common treatments offered for rheumatic and arthritic conditions, along with any possible side effects from their use, so that you are better able to discuss them with your doctor or recognize if they are suited to you.

Antibiotics

These drugs do not act directly on rheumatic or arthritic symptoms. Their function is to kill or slow the growth of bacteria which cause infection. Antibiotics are made from micro-organisms which have the ability to kill or slow the growth of other micro-organisms. They act upon either a wide range or a narrow range of bacteria or fungus. Antibiotics affect very few viruses and no antibiotic is a 'cure all'. They should be used strictly, as rarely as possible, and only after precise diagnosis of your problem. Not every infection should be treated with antibiotics because the body can handle most infection by itself. Over-use of antibiotics can create a resistance in the bacteria they are supposed to be killing. In other words, the antibiotic will no longer work and may, in some cases, cause further illness. Use of the wrong antibiotic may also create more problems than it solves. Antibiotics may have distressing side effects.

Osteomyelitis is generally caused by the staphylococcal infection and so it is treated, in part, with an antibiotic.

Rheumatic fever is sometimes treated with an antibiotic in order to prevent its reoccurrence. The antibiotic is chosen for its ability to kill the bacteria, not suppress their action.

Pott's disease and **Poncet's disease**, both caused by tuberculosis, are treated, in part, with antibiotics.

Infective arthritis is always treated with an antibiotic.

Antibiotics may also be given if a joint is to be drained of pus or fluid, or if open surgery is a necessary part of treatment.

The number of side effects from the use of antibiotics is increasing, as is the dangerous nature of these side effects. An antibiotic may kill off a nasty infection but, in doing so, it may allow other bacteria to flourish. These may well cause another, different infection in the body which may, in turn, require further drug treatment.

Such 'stacking' of illness is very hard on your body and it rapidly loses its resistance to bacteria that normally would not have presented any problem.

Some people are allergic to antibiotics and their reaction may be mild or severe, even fatal. Their reaction depends to some degree on how the antibiotic was given. For instance, given by mouth an adverse reaction may include nausea, vomiting or skin rash. Injected, a reaction may include kidney or liver damage, swelling, skin rash, fever and even anaphylactic shock (this is a severe allergic reaction which can be fatal). Side effects of antibiotic treatment, such as diarrhoea, do not always indicate an allergy. Skin rash however, is a common allergic reaction.

Antibiotics are often very effective but should not be used unless absolutely necessary and then under strict guidance from your doctor.

Braces, Supports and Appliances

Appliances are used to prevent deformity, to help relieve

pain, to support and protect an area of body while recovery takes place, and to help alter the function of muscles or joints. The most common and widely used treatment in this category is the simple practice of placing a board under the mattress, which helps to support your back during sleep. Even the firm cushion which you may position in your easy chair has remedial qualities if you suffer rheumatic discomfort.

Braces include splints and wired corsets. These are used to minimize or prevent movement of a painful and inflamed area so that pain and inflammation are reduced. This treatment is necessarily as short-term as possible in order that your muscles do not atrophy. Many find that relief is gained by using splints for the small joints at night only. Drug treatment often accompanies or follows the use of braces.

Supports include bandages, special shoes, pads or inserts. Their purpose is to minimize movement of a painful or unsatisfactory nature but not to prevent movement altogether. Use of supports encourages strength and elasticity in the muscles and ensures that the affected joint is used in the correct manner. Some support, such as bandaging, is best used in the short-term only. Other forms, such as special shoes, may be permanent or very long-term, perhaps while waiting for an operation.

Appliances include crutches, canes, walking frames and bed cradles. Their purposes are fairly obvious but, in general, they are not attached to the body and are used as accessories which enable safe movement and more rapid healing. A bed cradle is a frame which supports the bed clothes at night, to prevent the weight of blankets putting pressure on a painful area.

Drugs for Pain Relief

Also called analgesics, drugs which relieve pain often have the added effect of reducing inflammation and/or a fever.

Aspirin is a commonly used and readily available anti-inflammatory analgesic, relieving both pain and inflammation. Small doses (under 3 grams per day) help specifically to relieve pain but it is necessary to take over 3 grams per day in several small doses in order to reduce inflammation as well. (Maximum dose is 8 grams in 24 hours.)

Amounts over 3 grams can create problems in the stomach and intestines such as bleeding, ulcers, or nausea. Taking aspirin after eating will cut down on the amount of gastric discomfort suffered, but if you know you have gastric disorders, avoid taking aspirin.

Other side effects from aspirin include ringing in the ears, vertigo, and symptoms of allergy such as rashes, difficulty breathing and sharp pains in the chest. People who have allergic tendencies should avoid taking aspirin, as should those with kidney or liver problems. Pregnant and lactating women, the elderly and children under 12 years should also seek other treatment.

If you are already taking other drugs – especially diuretics, anti-coagulants, antacids, anti-epileptics or immuno-suppressants – please consult your doctor before using aspirin.

Paracetamol relieves pain and reduces fever, but has no anti-inflammatory effect. Maximum adult intake should not exceed 4 grams per day, taken in small doses.

This analgesic is less irritating to your stomach than aspirin, but it does cause liver damage if taken in overdose. This damage may not become apparent for 3–7 days. Alcoholics should avoid this drug.

Paracetamol should not be taken if you also take anti-coagulant drugs.

Colchicine relieves pain, specifically the pain of gout. It has a long history of use in the treatment of this ailment, but it should only be taken under your doctor's supervision.

Colchicine has toxic effects causing nausea, stomach pain, vomiting and occasionally rashes and diarrhoea. Pregnant or lactating women should avoid its use, as should the elderly and those with kidney, heart or digestive disorders.

Sedatives, though not generally prescribed to relieve pain, deserve some mention. One of the side effects of pain – in any disease – is a loss of positive outlook, possibly resulting in depression. As pain and loss of mobility become more dominant, so too might depression. At this point, you may feel overwhelmed and many doctors would prescribe a sedative to help you keep a sense of perspective.

Unfortunately, sedatives are generally addictive and they do not solve the problems which need to be confronted and resolved in order to maximize your health. It is wise to avoid them if at all possible. Lifestyle alternatives to sedatives are listed in chapter 6.

Drugs to Reduce Inflammation

Many anti-inflammatory drugs also relieve pain. Their effects on inflammation vary from person to person and your doctor may need to try several before one is found that is suitable. The anti-inflammatory drugs all have similar side effects which vary in intensity and great care must be taken to prevent serious complications.

In general, side effects include nausea, abdominal discomfort or bleeding in the stomach and intestines, although taking these drugs with food decreases the discomfort caused by them. A variety of further side effects can occur, including headache, ringing in the ears, vertigo, rashes and asthma, which indicate a hypersensitivity to the drug selected.

Pregnant women and those with kidney or liver disease should seek alternative treatment under medical supervision.

There are several NSAID's (non-steroidal anti-inflammatory drugs) available for use under prescription only and three examples follow:

Ibuprofen relieves pain and mild inflammation so it is useful in mild, chronic conditions and may be prescribed for children. People with a tendency to asthma or who suffer kidney, liver or stomach disorders should use this drug with caution.

Indomethacin relieves pain and mild or severe inflammation but should not be used by elderly people or pregnant women. Additionally, if you are epileptic, prone to allergy or asthma, or have liver or kidney trouble, avoid this drug. Cases of acute gout may respond to indomethacin.

Phenylbutazone is a very powerful anti-inflammatory drug which has recently been recommended for restricted use only by the Committee on Safety of Medicines. It is used for the treatment of ankylosing spondylitis, usually while the person is under hospital care. It is a drug best tried only if others do not help. Pregnant women should not use this drug and those with a history of liver, kidney, heart or thyroid disease should also avoid it.

Aspirin is still the most popular anti-inflammatory drug for regular use in rheumatic diseases. It is available without prescription but should be used sparingly and with full regard to its potential side effects.

Drugs to Reduce Your Fever

Both aspirin and paracetamol are useful to relieve fever. However, the Committee on Safety of Medicines has recently recommended that aspirin *not* be given to children under 12 years of age because of its possible contribution to Reye's syndrome, a rare condition which includes swelling of the brain and liver disorders, usually following a viral infection. Exceptions are in cases of juvenile rheumatoid arthritis, when aspirin may be given under doctor's supervision. Children may be given paracetamol instead in doses of:

60–120 mg for children under 1 year.
120–250 mg for children of 1–5 years of age.

43

250–500 mg for children of 6–12 years of age.

The most common side effects in adults are, from aspirin, irritation of the stomach and intestines and, from paracetamol, liver damage through overdose or prolonged use. Use both drugs *only when essential*.

Drugs Which Affect Your Hormones

Hormones are secreted into your blood by glands which are part of the endocrine system. Hormones are of many different types and have specific functions within the body including growth, metabolism, fertility – in fact, all of the body processes. Drugs are sometimes used to affect the action of hormones during rheumatic disorders. These drugs are themselves hormones, either extracts of a hormone or gland, or synthetic imitations of these hormones.

ACTH (Adrenocorticotrophic hormone) or **corticotrophin** is a hormone produced by your pituitary gland and it acts to stimulate your adrenal, thyroid and sex glands to produce their own hormones. When it stimulates your adrenal glands, a group of hormones is produced called corticosteroids, or sometimes just 'steroids'.

The **steroids** have become famous for their ability to reduce allergic and rheumatic reactions as well as inflammation. Their use has been modified since their 'discovery' because their powerful side effects have also become known. Now it is normal practice to use NSAID's (non-steroidal anti-inflammatory drugs), anti-inflammatory analgesics or anti-malarial drugs before resorting to a steroid.

Steroids do not cure; instead, they suppress the pain and inflammation of rheumatism and arthritis. While providing temporary relief, their use does not mean your problem is getting any better. Among the complications and side effects from use of steroids are dependence, retention of fluid and salt, loss of potassium, diabetes, osteoporosis, kidney stones, and retarded growth in children. The more severe of these side effects have been associated with specific steroids, such as hydrocortisone, and their use in general medicine has been greatly reduced.

The current use of hormone-linked drugs is confined to instances when other drugs do not prove effective. In such cases, it is preferable to have a local steroid injection directly into the inflamed joint or joints, or into the soft tissue surrounding – as in tendinitis. Both pain and inflammation are relieved as a result, therefore mobility is increased. **Prednisolone** is a steroid often used in this way as the dose can be finely adjusted to minimize side effects.

Drugs Which Affect Your Uric Acid Levels

An increase in the production of uric acid, or a decrease in its elimination from the body, results in uric acid salts depositing round the joints and in the kidneys. This causes gout, kidney stones, arthritis and the associated unsightly nodules or 'tophi' which may form, especially on the ear and fingers.

Anti-inflammatory analgesics such as indomethacin or colchicine are used to treat acute attacks of gout. Once the acute stage has passed, drugs which are used to control gout may be taken over an indefinite period of time.

A drug which reduces the production of uric acid is **allopurinol**. It is used only after an attack has passed, in order to prevent further attacks. It may cause digestive upsets, fever or even a rash and ought to be used along with an increased consumption of water.

Uricosuric drugs, such as **probenecid** and **sulphinpyrazone**, increase the excretion of uric acid. One of these drugs is used alone, or with allopurinol if the condition is stubborn. Plenty of clear fluids should be taken to help the excretion of the uric acid and frequent urination will, of course, result. Some digestive discomfort may occur, and possibly headaches, rashes or other signs of allergy.

These drugs should be used under doctor's supervision.

Drugs Affecting the Disease – Not Just the Symptoms

A group of drugs exist which are thought to slow, prevent or reverse the development of rheumatic disease. However, they are accompanied by powerful side effects and so their use is limited to those who have tried analgesic, anti-inflammatory and possible steroid treatment without success. Before using these drugs the rheumatic disease must have progressed over at least 6 months and after these drugs are introduced their effects may not be obvious for another 6 months. This time scale requires great patience. The underlying hope is that the disease will be slowed or stopped.

Gold (sodium aurothiomalate) is used in severe cases of RA, Still's disease or palindromic rheumatism. It is injected deep into the muscles about once a week to test for sensitivity such as skin rash or ulcers, then given in doses over a period of weeks until a total of 1 gram has been taken. The benefits of this treatment may take weeks or months to appear.

Chloroquine is an anti-malarial drug which is sometimes used as an anti-inflammatory treatment for rheumatism and arthritis. It is very powerful in its anti-inflammatory effect, but can cause damage to the retina of the eye, especially in older people whose eyes may be already weak.

Penicillamine is a drug normally of use in cases of

poisoning by metals. It works in a similar way to gold on both rheumatoid arthritis and Still's disease. It is taken in tablet form for one month to test for adverse effects and then the dose is increased gradually until the arthritis goes into remission. If there is no improvement within 12 months, the drug is discontinued. Some side effects to expect are rashes, especially in the early days of the treatment, temporary loss of taste and appetite, and nausea. It should not be used in company with other drugs, in the case of kidney disease or in pregnancy.

Immuno-suppressants or antimetabolites such as azathio-prine and methotrexate are used in cases where gold, penicillamine and chloroquine have proved unsuccessful. They may be used in company with steroids and have similar side effects, including nausea, diarrhoea and even vomiting. In some people, the herpes virus is made active during this treatment.

Counter-irritants
Ointments, liniments, packs and poultices are often applied to the skin to heat, irritate or cool the body surface. They are intended to relieve pain by creating a different sensation. Blood supply to the skin is usually increased, although this does not necessarily improve circulation to the deeper tissues. Change of temperature as well as counter-irritation do ease pain temporarily. Oils and liniments seem to work as a result of the massage which is used to apply them, rather than any pain-relief ingredients they might contain.

Rest and Immobility
All forms of rheumatism and arthritis benefit from rest. The exact amount of rest needed varies from person to person, and from one specific disorder to another. Rest is essential in order to keep your body refreshed and your mood positive. Up to ten hours of sleep in every day is worth aiming for, with brief periods of rest during waking hours. Too much rest, however, seems to create an 'invalid' or depressed state of mind which means you may lose the motivation to become well. Too much rest can also mean that mobility will be lost as a result.

In rheumatic and arthritic disorders pain and inflam-mation discourage movement, therefore a certain amount of determination is needed to prevent drastic loss of mobility. Regular exercises, however gentle, should become an essential part of your daily routine in order to maintain muscle tone and circulation to the afflicted area. If no exercises are done to prevent or minimize loss of mobility, the muscles around a joint will atrophy, joint destruction will occur more rapidly and, in some instances, osteoporosis may follow.

Surgery

In cases of an infected joint, tendon or bursa, surgery may be required. It will entail opening the area in order to drain pus and remove infected tissue. Infections which have progressed to the extent of killing bone – or in cases of bone 'chips' (called sequestra) spreading infection into the surrounding tissue – surgical removal of bone tissue is necessary.

Destruction of a joint may be treated by surgically replacing the joint (arthroplasty) to regain pain-free mobility or by pinning it (arthrodesis) to stop any movement of the joint. (See Osteoarthritis, chapter One.) This first operation is particularly common upon the hips which, being weight bearing, may cause severe pain and handicap if not treated. Joint replacement involves cutting the degenerated bone away and replacing it with a new joint made from synthetic material. Pinning a joint means inserting a metal pin between the two halves of the joint and then 'planting' bone chips – taken from some other part of the body – into the joint space. These chips produce more bone tissue which ultimately unites the pinned joint, rendering it immobile.

Both operations result in a pain-free joint and both require a positive frame of mind to ensure optimum recovery. Most important is that special exercises or physiotherapy be practised to build strength in the muscles and, in the case of pinning a joint, care must be given to correct posture and distribution of weight so that the other joints remain healthy.

More on possible side effects

Addiction, Dependence and Tolerance

These terms are often used interchangeably. Many drugs, when used repeatedly, create in you a powerful need to receive more of them. If this need is not met, you suffer physically and in many cases mentally also.

Specifically, **addiction** is used to describe a compulsive urge to obtain a drug and is usually associated with social and moral degeneration. Yet often addiction is induced without the subject's understanding or knowledge, as in use of sedatives. **Dependence** implies an emotional and mental need for a drug, whether or not it is accompanied by physical need. Some 'placebo' effect drugs have this result. **Tolerance** is generally used to describe your body's need for more and increased doses of a drug in order to induce the same effects a smaller dose previously had.

These side effects sometimes occur from use of drugs

intended to relieve the symptoms and discomforts of rheumatism and arthritis. The likelihood of suffering one of these side effects should be fully and clearly explained to you before treatment is begun.

Interaction with Other Drugs
If you do take drugs, it is rare for only one drug to be in use at one time. Your GP should ask you what drugs you already take regularly or even occasionally (such as contraceptive or headache pills) before prescribing a treatment for your particular disorder.

Depletion of Vitamins and Minerals
Most drugs exchange their particular action for some of your body's supply of nutrients. They don't simply add ingredients to your body, they use some up, too. Vitamins B, C and E are those most depleted when you use drugs – of any sort, coffee included. Of the minerals, calcium, zinc and iron are lost through regular drug use. Discuss your need for vitamin and mineral supplementation with your doctor if a drug is prescribed for your disorder.

Depression
The pain of your rheumatic disease is depressing in itself, especially if you have suffered over a long period of time. However, if you take drug treatment which robs you of essential vitamins and minerals you may slip further into depression – or experience it for the first time. This is an unfortunate side effect of both the disease and the drug treatment, one which should be confronted early on in your treatment.

If possible, avoid taking anti-depressants as they do not resolve either your disease or your nutritional deficiency. Instead, discuss alternatives with your doctor. A supplement or change of diet may be all you need. See chapters 4, 6 and 8 for other natural means of overcoming depression.

3

NATURAL
MEANS OF
OVERCOMING
RHEUMATISM
AND ARTHRITIS

**A General
Introduction
to Natural
Remedies**

There are three factors in any disease: 1) your physical symptoms, 2) your mental and emotional state, or background, and 3) the cause, or source, of your disease.

Take an example; imagine you have a bad cold. Your physical symptoms are runny nose and eyes, stuffed-up ears and waste-bins full of used tissues. Mentally and emotionally you may be in a sullen 'I want to be left alone' state. And no doubt the source of your cold was a germ which you picked up somehow and which decided to stay and create bother for you.

Why did it stay? Orthodox medicine understands the germ and the physical symptoms but doesn't always ask this question. It has named the germ and devised chemical means of suppressing the irritating symptoms it causes, but orthodox medicine does not necessarily discourage the germ from visiting you in the first place. It does not always prevent your body becoming a welcoming committee for that germ – whatever it is.

Natural medicine does ask the question – 'why did the germ stay?' It looks at all three aspects of disease at the same time, and the answer it finds is 'because you allowed it to stay'. Natural medicine looks at your symptoms, the germ itself and your mental and emotional condition (call this attitude). Then it treats your disorder so that all three factors are affected.

The result is often a mini revolution within your body, because natural medicine is not done *to* you, as orthodox medicine often is, it is done *with* you. Natural medicine cannot really happen effectively unless you become involved in your own treatment and begin to take responsibility for you own health – and your own disease. This is difficult, at first, for some people. But once you have won your first victory, and have begun to feel well through your own efforts with natural treatment, you will understand that responsibility can also bring a deeper respect for and understanding of your body.

Most natural medicines are based on an assumption that your body has an in-built capacity for creating and maintaining its own health. This is sometimes called integrity: that your body is complete and can meet all of its own needs *provided you allow it*. Natural medicine creates opportunity for this in-built capacity to work so that your body heals itself.

A deeper and longer term health is the usual result, a health that *prevents* your body welcoming all and sundry diseases. Because, after taking responsibility and trusting in your body's integrity, it is easy to include natural medicine in your daily life. In fact, it stops being 'natural medicine' and becomes, instead, just 'natural'.

What is 'Natural'?

Natural remedies are made up of the very basic substances which surround us – such as air, water, minerals and plants – together with our daily activities – such as diet, rest, elimination, thought and movement.

Natural remedies are those which do not intrude upon your state of health or add layers of confusion to symptoms of ill-health. They do not oppose you or your disorder, but work *with* nature to remedy health disorders at their source. And because the source, or cause, of illness can be attributed to virtually anything, so too remedies may arise from any of the natural substances which surround us.

When you use natural remedies to treat physical disorders, you create changes other than those of a purely physical nature. This is because natural treatment tends to view health in an 'all or nothing' manner. That is, if one part of you has a symptom of illness, *all* of you needs treatment, not just the one part. This is sometimes called a holistic view of health – where real health requires that your physical, mental and emotional aspects be 'balanced'. Natural remedies are more likely to be holistic in their approach to health because they aim to deal with the cause of disease, rather than only disguise it or relieve its symptoms.

Our world is itself becoming more diseased as we increasingly treat it in a less than wholesome or natural manner. So it is important to mention that natural remedies are best prepared using only those plants and minerals which are themselves healthy and as free from pesticides, chemicals and other adulterating agents as it is possible to obtain them.

Who Has Tried These Remedies?

Natural remedies are humankind's oldest, most successful and most established form of health treatment. Many of us are here now only because natural medicine worked for someone in our recent ancestry. Of course, some natural treatments did not work and our ancestors spent many generations learning, by trial and error, which treatments could be relied upon to remedy a disorder.

Some remedies have been successful for hundreds, some for thousands of years with variations only in their name, their presentation, or their availability – but not in their effect. Others proved unsuccessful and still others simply became unpopular as social and cultural priorities changed. So, for instance, it may be that chanting, shaking a rattle and dancing in a circle *is* an effective remedy for fever – but how would you react today to someone performing this ritual outside your door?

The remedies in this book are natural and well established. They have been tried and tested over generations of people and, while they don't all work for everyone, they have all worked for someone.

Is 'Natural' Better?

Not necessarily! If, for instance, you have very advanced osteoarthritis in one hip so that your life is painful and restricted, probably the best remedy is hip replacement surgery. This treatment will almost certainly give you pain-free mobility for a great many years – and a 'new lease on life' as well. But if your arthritis is not advanced, if you are waiting for an operation, or if you merely suspect that you may have a touch of arthritis, then natural treatment can be an effective and happy option.

Natural medicine aims to prevent or cure disease by treating it at source. Orthodox medicine also hopes to cure and prevent disease, but is increasingly caught up in relieving the symptoms of disease using unnatural substances. These substances tend to disguise disease and may create additional problems as a result, so that often more drugs are needed to relieve the new disorder!

In this respect, natural remedies can be safer than modern medical treatment. Most may be used over a very long period of time with only positive side effects because they are health-centred rather than disease-centred.

However, orthodox medicine is not your enemy. Your doctor wants you to be well and free from chemical bondage. Most doctors would rather not prescribe drugs unless they feel there is no alternative. And many doctors suggest natural forms of treatment in any case – diet, physiotherapy, exercise and stress reduction, to name a few.

Your doctor can become your best ally. You should aim to develop a relationship whereby he or she knows you want to be involved in your own treatment, but can give diagnostic and remedial advice – *both natural and orthodox* – as and when you need it.

Choosing a Remedy

Medical Diagnosis

Go to your doctor and have your problem diagnosed as soon after the appearance of symptoms as possible. By acting early, you may be able to prevent the disorder becoming very much worse. You will certainly be in a position to improve those aspects of your lifestyle, such as diet, rest and stress levels, which have an effect on the course of your disorder.

Some doctors state that diagnosis continues until you are well, by which they mean that your condition should be reassessed every time they see you. This does not mean, necessarily, that they will perform the tests or ask all of the questions as during your first visit. Diagnosis is really a continuous observation of symptoms and progress of disease in order that treatment may be sought. Your doctor may make an initial, general diagnosis and then, after learning more, make a precise one. Immediately a diagnosis is made, begin to discuss the range of treatment available to you. Especially tell your doctor that you are interested in using natural treatment as much as possible.

Reviewing What is Available
Come away from your visit with the name of your suspected disorder, the suggested remedy and as much information about both as possible. Now read whatever you can find regarding the disorder and the suggested remedy, including any side effects which may occur. Next, look into the natural treatments which are available and compare their effectiveness, safety and suitability with the orthodox treatments available.

Selecting a Remedy – Orthodox, Natural or a Combination
The treatment you select should be that which promises to be most effective in treating your disorder while causing you the least possible discomfort and addition of symptoms. However, your selection will also depend very much on how long you have suffered, how long you have used orthodox remedies, if at all, and how determined you are to feel as well as possible. Here are a few situations to illustrate the approach you may use:

● If, for instance, you have been suffering from osteo-arthritis for several years, chances are you have also been using drug treatment for nearly as long. You may be using a pain relieving drug during the day, as needed, and a sleeping pill at night because osteoarthritis can be particularly painful then. It is possible that, as a result of long-term use of such drugs, you will have acquired additional symptoms of ill health. These might include stomach pain or upset, ringing in the ears, and possibly dizziness – all from your use of pain relief drugs. You may be dependent on your sleeping pills – even if it is 'only' psychological dependence. And it is not uncommon, especially if you have changed doctors, to have been prescribed extra drugs to deal with these additional symptoms. So, you may be taking something for the dizziness, or stomach pains, as well as taking the drug that caused them in the first place!

The first step in resolving this very complicated network of symptoms is to take stock of precisely what drugs you use, how often you use them and how long you have been using them for. Include those which you buy over the counter and haven't necessarily been prescribed, such as aspirin. Then, either make a list of this information, or put the bottles and boxes in a bag, and make an appointment with your doctor. When you meet, show your list or the contents of your bag, say you are tired of feeling so many confusing symptoms and ask if he or she can sort the drugs into necessary and unnecessary.

Removing yourself from unnecessary drug treatment may take some time and you should follow the advice of your doctor as to the timing and order in which you stop taking them. You may find that, after several weeks or months, you have cut down on your drug treatment, feel very much better and are in a position to use natural remedies as part of your treatment. You will not only have improved your health but also clarified your disorder so that its cause can be treated.

● Here is another instance, this time assuming that your symptoms have appeared within the last two years. You will have probably visited your doctor at least once, have had some form of diagnosis and probably been recommended or prescribed treatment. You are in a position to use both natural and orthodox treatment if you choose, indeed, at this stage many doctors recommend fairly natural treatment in any case – such as exercise or change of diet. If your disease and your drug therapy is not very well established, you can consider the various treatments available for their long-term effects on you and your disorder. Your choice in the previous situation was limited in this respect because the disease and your drug history was already well established.

● The best position to be in (apart from in excellent health, of course!) is to have only recently experienced the symptoms of rheumatic disease and to be aware that you have a choice between natural and orthodox treatment. You may then receive a diagnosis of the symptoms and begin treatment fully aware of its likely advantages and disadvantages.

If you choose orthodox treatment, then educate yourself as to the safety and long-term effects of the drugs prescribed. If you choose natural treatment, be aware of the rate and pattern of improvement which is likely. And if you choose a combination of orthodox and natural treatment, be clear in your own mind as to why you are using each aspect of this combination.

Following the Treatment

Orthodox treatment requires that you act according to your doctor's instructions and supply him or her with information about your symptoms when necessary.

A combination of orthodox and natural treatment needs

you to understand the effects of each remedy you are using, for instance, the effects of your diet, your weekly massage and your monthly acupuncture session as well as your use of aspirin. If combination treatment is your choice, tell your doctor and describe which natural remedies you are using and why. Do your best to achieve a congenial relationship with your doctor so that he or she is able to understand and accept your wish for combination treatment.

Natural treatment used alone places you in a position of responsibility – your body gives you signals (symptoms) and you act on them by supplying treatment which you must also monitor yourself. Natural treatment leaves you the person most knowledgeable about and having most control over your own body in both health and illness. If you select natural treatment, please ensure that you:

a) retain a positive relationship with your orthodox medical doctor

b) attend only *qualified* natural medicine practitioners

c) learn as much as you can about health, nutrition and the remedies you use through reading, lectures, courses, and so on. If you are really committed to improving your health naturally, then you must become knowledgeable about all the fascinating aspects of your health and your treatment. Good Health!

There is a great deal of controversy as to whether or not diet is an important consideration in rheumatic conditions. Some within the medical profession proclaim adamantly that diet has nothing whatsoever to do with rheumatic disorders. Others keep an open mind, while still others are ·convinced that factors in your diet can cause, prevent and in some cases remedy rheumatic disease. But two aspects of the diet controversy are widely accepted within the medical profession.

The first accepted fact is that foods which contain a lot of purine should not be eaten if you are suffering from gout. Specifically, the organ meats such as kidneys and liver contain purine, a compound which your body changes into uric acid. The second accepted fact is that being overweight aggravates arthritic conditions – particularly of the large, weight-bearing joints. Your diet is therefore considered important in terms of weight reduction, if it is necessary.

Those who already suffer a rheumatic or arthritic complaint are often deficient in the B group of vitamins and they may suffer from constipation and/or hardening of the arteries. These conditions are readily improved through changes in the diet.

Foods to avoid in any rheumatic or arthritic condition are sugars, heavy fats such as butter, cream and fatty cheeses, meat – especially in cases of gout – coffee, alcohol and salty or heavily processed foods.

Foods to include are those rich in vitamins and minerals such as fresh fruits and vegetables, light oils, yogurt, yeast products – as in brewer's yeast or extract – and your favourite nuts and seeds (these latter tend to be rich in the B group of vitamins). In addition, plenty of clear fluids should be taken each day – up to about 12 glasses or cups. Clear vegetable broth, weak tea or herbal tea, water and fruit juices provide a pleasant selection.

Your diet may be used to counter the loss of vitamins and minerals incurred through the use of some drugs, such as antibiotics and sulphur drugs. You are particularly liable to be deficient in vitamins B and C if you rely on orthodox drug treatment.

Diet may also be used to bring about significant changes in the way your body deals with stress, toxins and infectious bacteria which are always present in our lives but need not always cause illness. Used in this way, diet is a preventative health measure.

'Diet' can mean a brief and temporary change of menu, or it can mean a completely new and long-term approach to your food and drink. The first implies equally brief and temporary benefits, the second implies a whole, vital outlook on life which results in improved long-term health. Here are some examples of diet treatments which may be of particular use in:

Gout	Osteoporosis
Infective Arthritis	Palindromic Rheumatism
Lumbago	Poncet's Rheumatism
Menopausal Arthritis	Pott's Disease
Neuritis	Rheumatoid Arthritis
Osteoarthritis	

Raw Juice Therapy

In this treatment the vitamins and minerals essential for health are supplied as much as possible through the consumption of raw juices, both fruit and vegetable. Because these foods are fresh and used in liquid form, they are easily digested and their nutritional value is readily available to the body. A regular intake of raw juices ensures that you get the vitamins and minerals you need and will gradually eliminate the deficiency-related disorders which accompany your rheumatic complaint. You may also find that this diet helps to relieve your pain. Improved health of the mucous membranes, muscle and bone tissue, digestion and elimination processes follow naturally from a diet of raw juices. You can look forward to greater mobility, more energy and a more positive outlook on life.

Fruits and vegetables selected for juicing are best if they are grown organically – without chemical sprays or fertilizers. If non-organically grown produce is used, the juice will contain concentrated doses of whatever chemicals were used in growing. These chemicals are toxic to the human body and will only complicate your attempts at becoming well. If you are uncertain about the growing conditions of the fruits and vegetables you select, put extra effort into washing or peeling them and try combining various juices. It is worthwhile purchasing a juicing machine if you intend to use raw juices on a regular or long-term basis. They make the juicing process quick and very easy.

A raw juice diet does not mean that juice is the only food taken. Instead, juice is made an important part of a diet which is light, balanced, varied and made up of unprocessed foods.

Here is an outline for a raw juice diet. Try it for one to two weeks and notice the difference in your health.

Begin the day by drinking a cup of hot water with the juice of half a lemon stirred into it. Lemon juice helps with digestion, elimination and weight loss and replenishes vitamin C in the body. Take the lemon juice dilution first thing in the morning, before you get out of bed if you can.

For breakfast select another fruit juice, such as apple. If you have a juicer you can get more adventurous and try cherry or strawberry juice instead. This drink should accompany a meal of toast or cereal with weak tea or herbal tea to follow. Avoid meat or fried foods.

Mid-morning, have another glass of fruit juice.

For lunch, have a large salad accompanied by a juice made from a vegetable such as carrot or beetroot. Some people prefer to combine vegetables in juice form – this is acceptable and very tasty. Carrot, celery and beetroot are excellent vegetables to use in a mixture. Other fruits and vegetables may be added to this 'cocktail' to suit your taste.

Mid-afternoon, take another glass of vegetable juice.

Your evening meal should exclude meat and fried foods. Instead, try eating another salad, perhaps with a soup starter. Drink a glass of vegetable juice before you eat.

At bedtime, drink a final glass of vegetable juice.

All of the food which you consume in the day should be fresh, unprocessed and low in salt, sugar and fat.

The value of various fruits and vegetables follows.
FRUITS

Apple: Rich in vitamin C, malic acid and a selection of minerals. This juice disinfects the digestive tract, prevents constipation and helps to remove toxins from the liver. A good juice to prevent complications in your health.

Cherry: Use up to ½ lb (225 g) of these daily to relieve gout. The juice acts on the digestion, liver and kidneys to clear uric acid from the body. Remove the stem and the stone before juicing.

Citrus: Oranges, grapefruit and lemons come into this category and they all have a cleansing effect on the intestines which prevents bowel disorders and problems with elimination. However, avoid grapefruit if you suffer from an ulcer or colitis. Orange and grapefruit should never be taken undiluted in arthritic or rheumatic cases as they can interfere with the absorption of calcium. Taken diluted just before a meal, they are very effective in killing off bacteria and stimulating the digestive process – especially useful if you are weak from pain. Lemon is the best juice to use on a regular basis as an early and mid-morning tonic. It does not interfere with the absorption of calcium.

Grape: High in iron and vitamins A, B and C, this juice is naturally sweet and therefore can be taken alone, in large quantities, over one or two days without causing weakness or loss of health. It prevents over-acidity in the body and helps in all forms of elimination and detoxification. Try this for gout or during acute rheumatic attacks.

Strawberry: Rich in vitamin C and high in iron and

calcium, this fruit makes a light and tasty juice. Strawberry juice is useful in cases of anaemia as its iron content is presented in combination with other nutrients to make the iron easy for the body to assimilate. Anaemia is very common if you are suffering an infection.

VEGETABLES

Beetroot: This juice is full of minerals that are presented in a way which makes them easy for your body to absorb. It removes toxins from the blood, increases the red blood cell count and reduces fever. In short, it is a real 'pick-me-up'. The juice may be combined with carrot or celery juice to enhance both its flavour and its healthy effects.

Carrot: Select the deep orange-coloured carrots which are better than the pale orange. This juice contains large quantities of Vitamin A, which benefits the pituitary, adrenal, and thyroid glands as well as the kidneys and liver. Carrot juice also keeps the mucous membranes throughout the body healthy and thus inhibits the spread of infection. Other benefits include good bone development and clear skin. This juice should be an important and regular part of your diet if you suffer a rheumatic complaint.

Celery: This juice is rich in minerals which have a soothing effect on the nerves and a stimulating effect on the major organs. In rheumatic and arthritic conditions it is used more specifically for its diuretic effect, which removes toxins from the body. Celery is rich in calcium.

Cucumber: Juice the whole of the cucumber, including the skin. It is valued for its diuretic property which is especially useful in some forms of rheumatism. Those who suffer high or low blood pressure as well as a rheumatic complaint will benefit from the high potassium levels in cucumber.

Dandelion: It is difficult for most people to find fresh, unsprayed dandelion leaves, but those who can should add the leaves to other vegetable juices. This plant has diuretic properties but, more importantly, it contains large amounts of vitamin A, calcium, magnesium and both sodium and potassium. This combination of minerals is of especial importance in the development and health of bone. Therefore, if you have disorders of the spine, osteoarthritis or any bone tissue disease, include dandelion in your raw juice diet.

Lettuce: Though not strictly a remedy for rheumatism or arthritis, the juice from this plant is exceptionally rich in minerals. For this reason it is a useful addition to your favourite vegetable juice. The outer, darker leaves, though usually less attractive, are more nutritious than the pale inner leaves.

Parsley: Another dark green leaf which is rich in vitamin A and generally high in mineral content. Parsley is good as an addition to other vegetable juices, adding a clean, earthy flavour. It acts as a tonic to the whole body, freshens the breath and is a mild diuretic.

Tomato: This juice is easily digested and supplies many of the essentials for general good health. Vitamins A, B, C, D and E are available in tomato, as are many minerals and trace minerals. Of course, fresh, raw and organically grown tomatoes are by far the most nutritious and tasty. This juice may be drunk by itself or mixed with other plants to make a juice cocktail.

Watercress: Add this to other juices or use it by itself in a dilution of mineral water. It is rich in minerals, particularly iodine, which benefits the thyroid gland. The main action of this juice is as a blood purifier – it removes toxins from the system and any beneficial effect on rheumatic conditions is due to this property.

NOTE: Do not mix grape juice with carrot juice or citrus juices with watercress juice.

Raw Foods Diet

A raw foods diet has been popular for generations as a way of improving and maintaining health. Many people have attributed drastic and immediate reversals in the progress of their disease to this diet. In fact, some of the healthiest and longest-living peoples in the world thrive on a predominantly raw food diet. The Hunza, a people who live high in the Himalayas, eat a diet of nearly 70 per cent raw foods and they are purported to be a culture 'without disease'.

There are two main benefits in following a raw foods diet. First, toxins are removed from the body rapidly and thoroughly. Second, the abundance of vitamins, minerals and trace elements present in raw food are easily assimilated by your body and quickly enhance your health. Here is a basic set of guidelines for your safe and successful use of an introductory seven-day raw food diet.

● You will need to 'book' one week (seven days) in your diary when you are not expected to go out to eat or to prepare an especially traditional meal. This precaution will make it easier for you to follow through with your diet, rather than having to explain or make special arrangements for raw food to be served for you. As this week approaches, do your best to clear temptation from your refrigerator and cupboards so that you are left with little or no food which is pre-cooked or processed.

● Instead, purchase raw fruits and vegetables daily to ensure maximum freshness and, when you can, buy organically grown produce to minimize the quantity of pesticides and other chemicals you take in with your food. As well as fruits and vegetables, you should choose a selection of nuts (if they 'agree' with you), seeds and grains. A wholefood shop will have a good stock to choose from. Look at the shopping list which follows.

Foods to Include in the Seven-day Raw Food Diet
Any raw, fresh fruit

Raisins, sultanas, prunes, figs, dates and other dried fruits *provided* they are sun-dried

Any raw, fresh vegetable – you *can* eat raw beetroot, turnip and cauliflower. Vegetables which need cooking, such as marrow, or that you do not find attractive in their raw state, should be avoided.

Raw, whole grains such as oat flakes, barley flakes, wheat bran and wheat germ. These may be mixed with fruit to form a cereal such as muesli, or sprinkled over a bowl of fruit to add bulk and vitamin value.

Raw nuts and seeds – avoid the roasted, dry roasted or heavily salted selections available and it is a good idea to avoid peanuts also if this is the first time you have tried a raw food diet. Instead, purchase raw nuts rich in vitamin B – such as brazil, almond, cashew, walnut, pistachio and filbert – and seeds such as sunflower, pumpkin, sesame, caraway and poppy. These are all tasty and nutritious with high vitamin and mineral values.

Cold-pressed olive or safflower oil

Fruit and vegetable juices, herbal teas and minerals waters

Honey

Plain, natural yogurt

Organic apple cider vinegar

Raw eggs – if you like them! Do limit your intake of these, however, as raw egg white reduces your body's supply of biotin, one of the B group of vitamins.

Wines from the Alsace region of France and other organic wines available in your local health-food shop.

Foods to Avoid in the Seven-day Raw Food Diet
Milk, cheese, butter, cream and margarine

Cooked eggs

Meat, fish and fowl and the fats from these animals

Bread, cakes, biscuits, crackers and pastry

Tinned and frozen foods and highly processed products such as breakfast cereals and snack foods

Sweets, chocolate, ice creams

Coffee, tea, cocoa, milk drinks, alcohol – apart from those organic wine varieties listed above

Any cooked or processed vegetables and fruit

Dried fruits which are not sun-dried – ask your shop keeper

Rice, millet, cous-cous, potatoes and all cooked grains and vegetables

Salt and sugar

You may be surprised to learn just how much of the food you normally consume is cooked in some way. By replacing it with totally raw food your vitamin and mineral intake will increase and the level of toxins in your system will decrease.

● This diet lasts seven days and during this time you should *eat as much food as you like.* Don't go hungry and don't feel that you have to abide by strict meal times or a limited intake of foods. If you feel as if you aren't getting enough food, eat more! Try a bowlful of sliced bananas and yogurt with a topping of oats and wheat germ, and when you make a salad, serve it up with an olive oil and cider vinegar dressing.

● If you are overweight, you can expect to lose some of it during this week, although that is not the purpose of this diet. Underweight people generally tend to eat more and feel brighter during this time – even if they do not actually gain weight.

● Depending on the level of toxins in your system, you may find that you develop a headache on the second or third day of this diet, or that a spot develops on your back or face. Both of these are signs that your body is getting rid of toxins, and perhaps knowing why they happen will make them easier to tolerate. The headache will go away – especially if encouraged by a cup of chamomile tea – and the spot will clear up. Just keep active and focus your thoughts on the positive outcome of the diet.

● *Do not continue this diet beyond seven days.* Instead, on the eighth day, begin to add healthy but cooked foods to your menu. (If you wish, you may repeat the seven-day diet again in six weeks.) Especially good are baked potato with a yogurt dressing, brown rice with steamed or raw vegetables, lentils and beans, wholewheat bread and yeast products such as marmite (yeast extract) and brewer's yeast. These foods are very nutritious and you should find them particularly tasty after a week of just raw foods.

● Flesh foods will not enhance your health and you should aim to cut them out of your diet entirely. Indeed, many people who have adopted a meat-free way of life for reasons other than health have reported that, as a bonus, their arthritis has disappeared. Flesh foods are difficult to digest, allow toxins to remain in the body and are low in essential vitamins and minerals. You will benefit more from experimenting with the great variety of other foods available to you. (See Appendix for list of meat-free recipe books.)

● *Do not stop eating raw foods entirely!* When you complete the diet, continue to eat plenty of salads, fruit and raw grains, nuts and seeds each day to keep the nutritional value of your diet high. This is most important if you are to take full advantage of the improvement in health brought about by your persistence in the seven-day raw food diet.

● What improvement should you expect? Well, for a start, your food will taste better and you will begin to enjoy it more. You will find that you have more energy and that your mood will be brighter. Also, you will feel less stiff in the mornings and – wait for it – you will probably feel less pain. People who have maintained a diet made up largely of raw foods have reported great improvements in their general health and, in some cases, a virtual disappearance of their rheumatic symptoms. This is because the food they eat is clean – it doesn't leave a lot of toxic material in the body – and highly nutritious, supplying the vitamins and minerals necessary for the body's systems to function at their best. For those many ailments and diseases which are caused or made worse by toxic matter in the body, this diet provides relief.

A Macrobiotic Diet

The guiding principle in macrobiotics is the presence of two opposite forces – yin and yang – in all things. These forces complement and balance one another. Based on ancient oriental philosophies, this concept has been popularized in the West, applied to food and given the name 'macrobiotics' by Mr Georges Ohsawa. Macrobiotics advocates a diet of in-season, whole foods which have been grown locally. But, there are no strict rules in the macrobiotic diet, only a firm contention that good health results from a balance of yin and yang in your diet and your life.

● The staple food of the macrobiotic diet is grain – rice, barley, wheat, rye, oats and millet. Pulses and lentils are also important, as are seaweeds and local fruits and vegetables. Meat, fish and dairy produce are avoided, as are coffee, tea and alcohol. Extreme foods such as sugar (extreme yin), salt and red meat (extreme yang) are also avoided.

● For the rheumatic or arthritic person, a macrobiotic diet can begin to undo the errors of a life of poor or inadequate diet by re-establishing balance. So, for instance, if you have always had a sweet tooth and now suffer from arthritis, it is possible that much of your problem can be eliminated by removing sugar from your diet – thereby adjusting the balance of yin and yang in your body. Similarly, if you have consumed large quantities of red meat, you may become unwell due to high concentrations of purine in your blood –

creating excess uric acid and all of its attendant problems such as gout and bursitis. Cutting out red meat and replacing it with grains and pulses will resolve this situation, your problem should improve and you will have adjusted the yin–yang balance in your diet.

● Mr Ohsawa recommends a strict, ten-day diet for those who truly want to rid themselves of their rheumatic disease. It is a simple diet: for ten days eat only unrefined whole grains. You may eat them raw, boiled, steamed, baked or fried. You may purée or cream them. Also, you may *eat as much as you like* provided you chew thoroughly. During this time, gradually reduce your intake of liquid, while avoiding tea and coffee. After the ten days you may gradually add lightly cooked vegetables, soups and fruits until you arrive at a diet you are happy with. If you follow this ten-day diet, then try also not to return to a diet high in sugar, meat, salt and fat.

● The health benefits of the macrobiotic diet include both prevention and cure, but there is usually a period of illness before either occurs. In a similar belief to naturopathy (see chapter 6), macrobiotics view illness as one way in which your body re-establishes health. In illness, the body releases the toxins or the stress which has caused your illness in the first place. If this is allowed to happen, without the intervention of drug therapy, then the illness will run its course quickly and your body will be left 'clean' and well. This approach frightens some people who do not believe in their body's ability to heal itself, especially as an illness left untreated by drugs may appear more severe than one prolonged – but suppressed – by drug therapy.

● The macrobiotic diet gives you a background of health which improves as the diet becomes a way of life. You gradually gain an understanding and confidence which enables you to respond, through your diet, to the needs and demands of your life and your environment. (See Appendix for further reading.)

Eating Without Allergy

Food allergy is often called food intolerance and it is generally believed that the potential for it is founded in infancy. During this vulnerable time, foods may be introduced into your diet for which you are not yet ready. At this time, and later in life too, your body may be unable to digest these foods fully and so the undigested particles are treated as foreign and unwanted by your immune system. The 'attack' response which follows is the same as that which occurs when you suffer from a virus, for instance. Instead of recovering, however, if you continue to eat the food which initiates the immune response, you will continue to suffer symptoms of illness. Most food intolerance suffered in this way causes very obvious and immediate reactions such as rash, migraine or diarrhoea and you usually stop eating that food as a result.

However, if the symptoms are not at first obvious, you might continue to eat the food and so acquire symptoms of illness more gradually. Food intolerance which develops gradually is very common and is thought to be the cause of many of the chronic diseases we suffer from – rheumatism and arthritis are an example.

Unfortunately, some foods are now so chemicalized (pesticides, fertilizers, fungicides) that it is difficult to know whether you have a *food* intolerance or a *chemical* intolerance. Try buying organically grown fruits, grains and vegetables – they are grown without chemicals and you will know from eating them where your intolerance lies.

Here are some preliminary steps you can take to determine whether, and which, food may cause your disorder.

How to Find the Foods You Do Not Tolerate

It may seem odd, but – apart from obvious and immediate reactions like skin rash – food intolerance is often felt as food addiction. For instance, if you have strong and regular cravings for chocolate or bread, you are probably also intolerant of them. They may be contributing to your eczema, your asthma or your arthritis without you having noticed. How do you find out for sure?

● Note whether you seem to need those foods when you are under stress for any reason.

● Note also whether you eat them daily, at least once, without fail.

● Note whether eating them makes you feel very much better, even elated.

If you observe these tendencies in yourself, suspect a food allergy.

● The final test is simple: eliminate that food from your diet for 24 hours. If you get a headache then you have some intolerance of the food. And, just to be sure, eat a little of it; if your headache disappears you know that the food is creating problems for you.

There are food intolerances which are commonly associated with rheumatic and arthritic disorders. Some are listed here for your information. You may find that none of them create any problems for you, or that one or two contribute to your symptoms.

Eggs	Milk
Soya beans	Beef
Yeast	Chicken

Peanuts	Potatoes*
Tomatoes*	Aubergine*
Tobacco*	Peppers*

Note that five members of the nightshade family of plants (asterisked) are included in this list. If you find you are sensitive to one food from this family, try eliminating the others from your diet also.

How to Eliminate the Food from Your Diet

If you suffer immediate symptoms of allergy to a food, then you probably don't eat it in any case. But if yours seems to be an allergy with 'quiet' or gradual symptoms, then you will need to make an effort to eliminate that food from your diet. There are several ways of doing this.

● You can simply stop eating it. If you choose this method, please do so with the knowledge of your GP because this is a traumatic event for your body. Up until now you have been giving your body regular doses of a food which it finds intolerable, yet has come to depend upon. When you stop giving the doses, you will probably have to endure headaches, tiredness, aching muscles and joints, nausea, irritability and depression or any number of other uncomfortable symptoms of withdrawal. You will not feel well and you may feel awful. The good news is that it doesn't last for ever.

You may get by with a mild version of withdrawal symptoms, or you may have to put up with them for several days. But when your withdrawal from that food is complete, you will also have cleared your body of the stress and toxins which eating the food created. What you will notice then is less fatigue, less stiffness, fewer aches and pains.

● You may *gradually* eliminate your intake of that food. This method has the same final result as the previous method, but without the trauma. You may feel less energetic and less well than 'normal', but you will not suffer unduly from the removal of toxins which have accumulated in your body. Allow yourself a week or two to cut out your consumption of that particular food by eating less and less of it each day.

● Finally, you may reduce the amount of that food in your diet. In this method, you need not aim to eliminate it completely from your diet. Instead, make certain that you eat it only once or twice each week and then in small quantities. This level of consumption is suitable only if you do *not* suffer strong withdrawal symptoms when you do not eat that food.

Recognizing and dealing with food intolerance is a very personal matter and, although you may wish to consult a doctor or a specialist in allergy, you are usually the first person to know how you react to the foods you eat. That puts you 'in the driving seat' with responsibility for observing what you eat, how you eat it and how you react to it.

A Vegetarian Diet

Many studies now indicate that an emphasis on non-animal sources of protein in your diet can benefit your health. There are several reasons why this may be so and, in particular, why a vegetarian diet can improve your rheumatic complaint.

There are 'layers' within the vegetarian concept. Some people call themselves vegetarian but still eat fish, others eat eggs and milk products but no fish and call themselves 'lacto-ovo vegetarians'. And still others, vegans, eat no animal produce whatsoever. *Any* reduction in the amount of animal produce you consume will benefit your health.

When you eat flesh foods you body must work very hard to process them. It takes nearly twice as long for your body to digest meat than to digest plant foods. That means that all the waste products which naturally result during the digestive process remain in your body and become quite toxic. And as we know, toxins which are not readily expelled from your body can contribute to disease, pain, inflammation and general loss of health.

Flesh consumption ensures that large, even excessive, quantities of fat are taken into your system. And digesting fat is a very stressful activity for your body. Especially if you are already overweight, fat contributes to the disorders – such as circulatory, kidney, liver and heart problems – which often accompany and aggravate the rheumatic diseases.

Finally, when you eat animal produce regularly, you are less likely to consume adequate amounts of plant foods which supply the range of vitamins and minerals so essential to health. You are also liable to leave yourself in very short supply of fibre in your diet – after a meat meal there just isn't enough room! You are therefore vulnerable to gross deficiencies in your diet as well as to chronic constipation. Again, the result is additional stress for your body and a larger collection of companion disorders to your rheumatic disease.

A diet low in, or devoid of, animal products is easy and exciting to achieve. If you allow yourself a few months to make the switch, and maybe treat yourself to a vegetarian cooking course, you can ensure that you are not left confused or hungry by your new diet.

In fact, many people naturally 'go off' meat products as they get older and some describe leaving meat out altogether as a positive relief! Certainly, the nutritional value of your diet will increase if you replace animal products with plant foods. Almost certainly, your rheumatic disease will lessen its grip on your life.

The Yogurt Programme

This is a way of minimizing some of the side effects of drug therapy. Assuming that you are, or have been, taking antibiotics or sulphonamides, you may suffer from loss of appetite, nausea, diarrhoea or headache. This usually occurs because these drugs can kill off some of the useful bacteria in your intestines (as well as the not-so-useful) which normally help you to digest your food.

Fresh, natural yogurt, if eaten regularly, can reinstate bacteria which are important for proper digestion. These bacteria prevent your food from loitering in your intestines and becoming toxic, and therefore improve your ability to digest food and absorb all of its nutrients. The best yogurt is that which is made from lactobacillus acidophilus. This is a micro-organism which, when introduced to milk, causes it to ferment changing the lactose in cow's milk, for instance, into lactic acid. Goat's milk and soya milk may also be used to make yogurt. The lactobacillus acidophilus is available from most health food shops. (If in doubt, why not try making it yourself?) Any unsweetened, unflavoured yogurt, however, will help you to resolve digestive problems such as those caused by the use of antibiotics and associated drugs. Try eating 4–10 oz (100–275 g) of natural yogurt daily for your good health.

Eating for Weight Reduction

Being overweight can aggravate the symptoms of a rheumatic disorder. In particular, those who are afflicted in the weight-bearing joints of the body, i.e. the hips, knees and lower back, will suffer more if they are overweight. In such cases, weight reduction is a first step in minimizing discomfort and improving overall health. Some surgeons require especially obese persons to lose weight before they will even consider performing an operation such as a hip replacement.

Excess weight is hard on the body. It causes stress and complications – in all of the body's systems – which gradually undermine health. It may also make treatment of illness, any illness, more difficult because of the effect of drugs, therapy or surgery on an already overworked body.

How do you tell if you are overweight? There are charts in most doctors' surgeries and in many books on nutrition which describe an ideal weight for your height and sex. These are useful as approximate guidelines, but you probably know already whether or not you are overweight – and if you are it is in your interest to lose weight as part of a health 'insurance' plan. It is also important that you take a responsible and long-term view of weight management right from the start.

It is possible to eat very well *and* lose weight by eating only those foods which supply vitamins, minerals and essential nutrients, but not surplus calories. Rather than adopting the 'dieting' approach of 'not eating', which robs you of nutrients as well as calories, you can eat your fill of healthy, nutritious, low-calorie foods and lose weight while you gain health. Eating for weight reduction is a positive approach to long-term health. Selecting food for its nutrient value begins to restore your health and, if continued, will maintain your health at its optimum.

A basic, healthy diet for weight reduction may be derived, in part, from the raw juice and raw foods diets listed above. Raw, fresh and unprocessed selections from each of the fruit, vegetable, nut, seed, legume and grain groups of food should comprise a large part of your daily diet. Here is a sample menu:

Breakfast:
Fresh fruits with yogurt *or*
Muesli with yogurt, soya milk or fruit juice, *or*
Toasted wholewheat bread with honey or yeast extract *and*
Fruit juice, herbal tea or mineral water

Mid-morning:
Weak tea, herbal tea, fruit or vegetable juice *and*
Raw fruit or vegetable (i.e. apple, carrot, celery, banana)

Lunch:
Fruit or vegetable salad with yogurt or lemon juice dressing *and*
One slice of wholewheat bread *and*
Mixed nuts, seeds and dried fruit snack *and*
Weak tea, herbal tea, fruit or vegetable juice

Mid-afternoon:
Weak tea, herbal tea, fruit or vegetable juice *and*
Raw fruit or vegetable *or*
Mixed nuts, seeds and dried fruit snack

Dinner:
Salad starter *and*
Light soup or broth *and*

Baked potato with steamed broccoli *and*
Steamed carrots, butter beans or green beans *and*
Yogurt and fresh fruit *and*
Herbal tea

While you are eating for weight reduction maintain a calorie intake of *at least* 1500 per day to keep your health. In fact, after the first week or two, try to do away with too much calorie counting – it can be extremely stressful in itself. The point is to gain health, not to worry. And don't go hungry! Raw foods tend to supply fewer calories than processed foods so if you feel peckish eat something raw. Eat as much raw food as you like, whenever you like and, if possible, buy organically grown fruits and vegetables. Remember, you are eating to gain health as much as to lose weight, so select your food for its health value and the pounds will start to roll off.

Supplementing Your Diet Naturally

In an ideal world, the food you eat should provide you with all of the nutrients necessary to maintain good health. Your body was designed to take food, not supplements, and it is far better for you to correct and improve your diet before turning to dietary supplements. Without a doubt, they are costly. In addition, their effects are difficult to measure because there are so many variables both in the manner in which they are taken and in the precise composition of the thousands available on the open market.

However, poor quality food, a diet without much variety or a diet that does not supply enough food can leave you deficient in one or more essential vitamins and minerals. Also, previous illness or injury may have left you unable to assimilate your food as well as you should. In these cases, it may be possible to make up deficiency by adding substances to your diet which, while they may not supply you with calories, contribute to your stores of vitamins and minerals. These substances are called supplements. They should not replace food in your diet; instead, they are intended to enhance your diet and to counteract the detrimental effects of drugs, stress and other environmental conditions upon your health.

If you have suffered ill-health for a long time, are recovering from an operation, or if you know that your food does not supply enough nutrients because of the chemicals used in growing and preserving it, then you have valid reasons for supplementing your diet *provided you have tried to improve the quality of your diet first*. It remains to decide what form of supplementation is best suited to you.

The examples that follow are supplements commonly

used by those who suffer from rheumatic disorders, in particular:

Dry joint	Menopausal arthritis
Fibrositis	Osteomyelitis
Gout	Rheumatoid arthritis
Lumbago	Tendinitis

Alfalfa Alfalfa is also called lucerne (*Medicago sativa*) and is a member of the legume family. It is rich in protein, minerals – especially calcium – and fat-soluble vitamins (A, D, E, F and K). The chlorophyll which alfalfa contains is a very potent, natural detoxifier acting through the kidneys. A detoxifier releases various toxic substances from where they are stored in the fatty tissues around your liver, kidneys, heart and muscles. These substances are pushed into your bloodstream and from there excreted from your body through perspiration, urine, waste and breath. Alfalfa is particularly good at the detoxifying process and it affects rheumatic disorders by reducing the pain and swelling which accompany toxic accumulations. In some people pain and inflammation disappear altogether.

Alfalfa is sold as tablets, powder and tea. The tablets are available in a fibre-free form so that their action is based entirely on the protein, vitamins and chlorophyll which remain. Follow the manufacturer's instructions for dosage. A largely raw foods diet should be practised once initial improvement has been achieved.

Ginseng This is a common name for a plant (*Panax quinquefolium*) whose root has been used for thousands of years in the Far East as a preventative medicine in all diseases which affect the endocrine (lymph) system. Rheumatoid arthritis, gout and lumbago are among those disorders which ginseng is said to treat, especially if taken regularly.

Ginseng stimulates the glands which control your body's metabolism and is purported to improve your resistance to illness and fatigue. However, there is no proof that this is so. Ginseng does contain vitamins and trace minerals which may improve your body's ability to assimilate the vitamins and minerals present in your food.

Sold in the form of capsules, ginseng is often recommended to elderly people who may have lost strength in their muscles as it is thought to stimulate the formation of new muscle tissue, thus reducing the likelihood of atrophy in those whose movement has been impaired.

Please use this supplement with care and, if you have kidney or liver problems, consult your doctor or natural medicine practitioner before taking it.

Honey and Cider Vinegar

Dr D. C. Jarvis, from Vermont in the USA, popularized this remedy through the publication of his books illustrating its effect on various disorders (see Appendix). Both cider vinegar and honey have a high mineral content which includes calcium, phosphorus, sodium and potassium, iron, copper and zinc. Traces of the B group of vitamins as well as vitamin C are present in some brands of cider vinegar.

Apart from supplying valuable minerals, honey and cider vinegar alter the acid/alkali balance in the body so that many disorders such as hypertension, colds and flu, migraine, skin problems, digestive upsets and, of course, the rheumatic diseases are discouraged.

Honey and cider vinegar is of particular use in cases of fibrositis, gout, osteoporosis, rheumatoid arthritis and tendinitis. Here's how it works:

The cider vinegar helps your body assimilate calcium (see separate entry on Calcium, this chapter). It does this by creating hydrochloric acid in your stomach (a natural acid, already present in the stomach) so that any calcium taken in your diet is dissolved – then either made use of, 20–30%, or excreted 70–80%. This is what *should* happen with calcium in any case, but in some people – even though they take adequate amounts of calcium in their diet – the body does not assimilate it because there is insufficient acid. Instead, the calcium is deposited in the joints, arteries and muscles. This can mean that the person is actually left *deficient* in calcium, but suffers the pain which accompanies calcium build-up in the joints and soft tissues.

You can see how this can be both confusing and frustrating to someone who does their best to eat a calcium-rich diet. Calcium deposits already present in the joints, muscles and arteries are also gradually dissolved by a supplement of cider vinegar in the diet and pain is greatly reduced or eliminated as a result. Also, disorders which often go hand in hand with rheumatism, such as constipation, varicose veins, digestive problems and so on, are usually improved with the use of honey and vinegar.

The remedy is most effective if you begin using it early on, as soon as, or even before, you notice symptoms of a rheumatic condition. It is popular because it has been very effective in reducing pain, stiffness and swelling – even in those who do not alter their diet in any other way.

The 'dose' used in this remedy is one tablespoon each of cider vinegar and honey stirred into a cupful of warm water. This amount is taken three times daily: once on rising, once after lunch and once before bed.

Kelp

Kelp is a seaweed which grows in strands up to 100 ft (30 m) long in kelp beds off the coasts of Ireland, France, California and Japan. It has been included in the local diets for generations and is responsible for the sometimes surprising good health of the coastal people. Kelp contains large quantities of vitamins B, D, E and K as well as calcium, potassium, magnesium and iodine – in fact, about fifteen minerals in total. It is considered to be the best source of natural, organic iodine which is essential for the production of hormones in the thyroid glands. If you recall, these hormones influence your metabolism and the way your body functions in both illness and health. A hormonal imbalance instigates rheumatic disorders in many cases – through stress, emotional trauma, chemical poisoning – and kelp may help to prevent or minimize this dysfunction.

Kelp as a supplement to your diet is available dried, powdered or in tablet form and should be taken regularly. If you do not like taking tablets, try sprinkling the powder on a piece of toast or into a salad dressing. Dried strands of kelp may be used in soups, stews or casseroles to make a thick, delicious and health-giving stock.

Sarsaparilla

Sarsaparilla has tonic and blood purifying properties which make it a useful remedy in rheumatic conditions, especially if a healthy diet is followed at the same time. The root is powdered, an extract taken from it or a syrup made for dilution. For regular use, two tablespoons of syrup in ½ pt (300 ml) of water makes a very tasty and refreshing drink for mid-morning or mid-afternoon.

Sarsaparilla also acts upon the production and synthesis of hormones in the body, and does itself contain hormones similar to those secreted by your adrenal gland. Your body needs these hormones in order to maintain its defences against infection and to prevent general malaise. If, due to sluggish metabolism, previous ill-health or prolonged use of drug therapies, their production is impaired, you become more susceptible to chronic disorders. Sarsaparilla is a possible means of correcting this shortage and, at the same time, supplies your body with minerals essential to keeping the health you have gained.

Sarsaparilla is found in a number of anti-rheumatic herbal treatments where it is usually included for its cleansing and tonic effect.

Vitamins and Minerals

Your body requires several dozen nutrients in order to remain healthy. When they are not supplied in your diet, illness usually results because poor nutrition causes stress in the body, making all of its normal functions more difficult. If this is the only source of stress, then a change in diet will quickly remedy the problem. Often, however, many other factors create stress, among them fatigue, anxiety, over-work, lack of exercise, infection, injury, or environmental pollution.

All of these sources of stress increase your body's need for the vitamins and minerals that maintain good health. But, sadly, most of us do not increase our supply of these nutrients at stressful times and the result is deficiency, more stress and an even greater likelihood of illness. And by the time illness has shown all of its symptoms, you may have begun to use drugs and other forms of treatment which can further reduce the supply of essential nutrients to your body. This is a vicious circle which is easy to fall into: treating the signs of deficiency with drugs which increase the deficiency rather than remedy it.

Vitamin and mineral supplements are intended to help slow and ultimately reverse deficiency when ample nutrients are not supplied through a varied, natural diet. When you don't know for certain how nutritious your food is, have eaten largely processed food or used drug therapy for a long period of time, a vitamin and mineral supplement may be a good investment. Here are the main nutrients needed for health, especially in people who suffer from a rheumatic or arthritic condition. All of these are available in supplement form and are most valuable if made from pure and natural, rather than synthetic, ingredients.

NOTE: Fat-soluble vitamins are stored in the body and so you do not need to take great quantities of them on a regular basis. Your body uses its store of these vitamins as and when it needs. Water-soluble vitamins are not stored and may be taken frequently as any surplus is passed from your body.

VITAMINS

● **Vitamin A** is a fat-soluble vitamin which is present in two forms: carotene and pre-formed. Carotene is available in a great many foods such as carrots, spinach, broccoli and other dark green, leafy vegetables. The body converts some of the carotene in these vegetables into preformed vitamin A, which is stored in the liver, kidneys, lungs and eyes.

Vitamin A is necessary for the formation of strong bones and teeth, good eyesight and digestion and healthy skin. The mucous membranes throughout the body are kept in good health with adequate supplies of vitamin A and these membranes help to prevent infection. Indeed, this is perhaps A's most valuable function in the person suffering from rheumatism because infection is often either the cause of, or a complication to, their problem.

A deficiency in vitamin A may also create a vitamin C deficiency.

● **Vitamin B** is really a group of vitamins, often called the vitamin B-complex. It consists of more than twelve different water-soluble substances which appear in many foods such as green vegetables, nuts, seeds and whole grains and can also be derived from fungi, mould or yeast. A member of the B-complex never appears in isolation in a food – and never acts in isolation either. The B vitamins need each other in order to function as they should upon the body, so if one is taken in isolation a deficiency in another member of the group will usually result. For this reason, it is best to obtain your supply of the B-complex from your diet, because the B's are presented as a group in your food. However, if you know your food is of poor quality or that you are already deficient in the B-group, you should take a natural vitamin B-complex supplement (usually derived from yeast). And if you decide to take one member of the B-group, for instance vitamin B6, by itself you should take a B-complex supplement at the same time to prevent any deficiency occurring.

Alcohol, sugar, coffee, stress of any sort, trauma and the normal metabolic processes of digestion and growth increase your body's need for the B-group of vitamins. If you suffer from a rheumatic disease and also take drugs to relieve its symptoms, you are greatly increasing your need for vitamin B and should improve or supplement your diet. Similarly, if you feel worn down and generally unwell from the rheumatic condition you suffer. Allergic symptoms, whether to drugs or foods, may be minimized by a regular intake of the B-group of vitamins, which also affect the functioning of your adrenal glands. Your digestive and endocrine systems, nerves and skin will all benefit from adequate vitamin B in your diet. Any surplus is eliminated from your body.

Many women fall prey to the rheumatic family of diseases in their childbearing years. Women of this age should endeavour to eat foods high in the B-complex and to supplement their diet with vitamin B tablets or liberal amounts of brewer's yeast.

● **Vitamin C** is another water-soluble vitamin which is most crucial for the formation of strong cells. In rheumatic disorders, vitamin C is necessary to prevent excessive swelling, bleeding and pain which can be caused by the breakdown of red blood cells. High levels of vitamin C (also called ascorbic acid) in your blood thins the fluid in your joints, making it easier for you to move. In addition, this vitamin enhances your body's ability to use the B-complex and vitamins A and E.

Fresh fruits and vegetables, especially with a deep red or green colouring, are excellent sources of vitamin C and these should be eaten daily as vitamin C is not stored in the body for longer than three or four hours. It is best to obtain the necessary supply of this vitamin from your diet when possible and to 'top up' during stressful times with a dietary supplement.

Illness, infection, smoking and the use of drugs ranging from aspirin to cortisone all increase your body's need for vitamin C. If it does not receive enough of this vitamin, you will begin to notice more pain and inflammation of the joints, you will bruise easily and heal slowly. You will also be more susceptible to colds and infections and you will begin to feel generally 'run down'. Your need for vitamin C increases with age and, especially if you suffer from arthritis, rheumatism or any chronic disorder, a regular supplement taken with a healthy diet may well prevent severe deficiency and further complications in your health.

Vitamin C should be taken in small, frequent doses (approximately 250 milligrams three to six times daily) on a regular basis and, in times of special need, this amount may be increased.

● **Vitamin D**, a fat-soluble vitamin, is known as the sunshine vitamin because the sun reacts with a substance in your skin, dehydrocholesterol, to make vitamin D. Most people can, with normal exposure of the sun, derive adequate supplies of vitamin D for their health. In your diet, this vitamin is derived from 'fortified' products, particularly milk products. Supplements of vitamin D are only of use when calcium and phosphorus are present in adequate amounts in your diet as these three substances act together. Vitamin A also acts with vitamin D.

Your body's ability to assimilate and transport calcium and phosphorus is dependent on supplies of vitamin D, and normal bone development is a result of this process. Usually associated with childhood growth and, in deficiency, with rickets, vitamin D is also necessary to prevent disorders related to calcium loss. You should discuss with your doctor whether or not you need a vitamin D supplement. People with dark skin, especially pregnant women, may need vitamin D supplements as high pigmentation produces less vitamin D.

● **Vitamin E** is fat-soluble and available in wheat germ,

vegetable oils, seeds, nuts and beans. It enhances the action of other major nutrients by preventing them from breaking down before your body can use them. This is called oxidation, therefore vitamin E is an anti-oxidant. It is essential in the process of nourishing and preserving the health of cells – blood and lymph especially – and is important in cases of arthritis, bursitis and gout where the health of the blood and lymph affect the severity and progress of the disease.

Supplementation of your diet with vitamin E may well improve general health as well as rheumatic conditions. This is because it acts on most of the body tissues through the blood and lymph. Vitamin E may be taken daily in one dose of 15–100 IU's (International Units). If you also take an iron supplement, take it at the opposite end of the day from this vitamin.

MINERALS

● **Calcium** is essential to the formation and maintenance of bones and teeth. Surprisingly, you need more as you get older because your body's ability to absorb it decreases with age. Calcium is present in milk, cheese, soya products, seaweed, dried fruits, almonds, celery, dark green leafy vegetables, kale and a great many other delicious foods. For maximum benefit, calcium foods are best eaten separately from starchy food. Also, avoid chocolate, rhubarb and spinach if you have a calcium deficiency.

Only about 25 per cent of the calcium you take in is absorbed by your body and other nutrients affect this rate of absorption. Phosphorus is perhaps the most important of these, although magnesium and vitamins A, D and C are also crucial. It is best to derive these nutrients from your diet. However, if a deficiency exists a supplement may be taken.

Osteoporosis, arthritis, fibrositis and many of the companion disorders to rheumatic conditions can be improved through adequate and accessible supplies of calcium. In supplement form, 800–1200 milligrams daily is the recommended dose when accompanying a healthy, fresh food diet.

● **Magnesium** helps your body make use of minerals and vitamins and, in general, plays a crucial role in how your body metabolizes. The B-complex, vitamins C and E, calcium, phosphorus and both sodium and potassium are all affected by the quantity of magnesium in the body. Therefore, magnesium is important in the development of bones, teeth, muscle and nerve, and in all of the basic life processes which require these nutrients.

In your diet, magnesium is present in nuts and seeds, fresh green vegetables, fruit and soya beans. Your body usually absorbs the magnesium it requires from your diet; however, if you are using a diuretic or a hormone drug or consume a lot of alcohol, you would do well to supplement the magnesium in your diet. Approximately 300 milligrams per day, in total, is the recommended intake of magnesium – whether from your diet, from supplementation, or from a combination of diet and supplements. This mineral is usually present in the multi-mineral tablets currently on the market.

● **Potassium** is a mineral which works together with sodium to keep the fluid (water) inside and outside the cell walls in balance. Your heart, nerves, kidneys and skin especially rely on an adequate supply of potassium, but all metabolic processes require that it be present in balance with sodium. Magnesium helps maintain correct levels of potassium.

Potatoes and bananas provide excellent sources of potassium, with oranges, sunflower seeds and green, leafy vegetables also containing useful quantities. Alcohol, sugar and coffee deplete supplies of potassium as does a high intake of salt (sodium).

● **Phosphorus** is present in every cell in your body. It works with calcium to develop bones and teeth and to maintain them in good repair. This mineral is important to the contraction of muscles – even those you don't see, such as the heart – and is used in nearly every function your body performs.

A deficiency of phosphorus leaves you feeling tired, nervous and with too little or too large an appetite. Prolonged deficiency can cause stunted growth, bone deformation, tooth decay and arthritis. Phosphorus is found in eggs, seeds, whole grains and nuts. You need to have calcium and vitamin D in adequate supply to ensure that phosphorus will be absorbed from your diet. A high-fat or high-sugar diet will reduce the amount of phosphorus you are able to absorb and these excesses should be avoided.

5

EXERCISE

AND THE

OUTDOORS

Have you heard this old saying? 'If you don't have time for exercise, you'll certainly have time for illness.' This applies especially if you suffer from a rheumatic disorder.

There are many physical benefits to be gained from regular exercise. Exercise keeps your muscles supple and strong so that they support your joints, it helps to prevent loss of mobility and joint destruction, and increases circulation throughout your body. Exercise also stimulates the circulation of lymph, thus reducing inflammation and removing toxic substances from your body. These benefits result in improved overall health and a more active and pain-free life if you have a rheumatic complaint. There are certain guidelines to follow, however, if you want to ensure that your exercise is safe, effective and beneficial.

If you exercise, you must also rest – and vice versa. You should not have one without the other. If you rest too much, your muscles atrophy, your joints become rigid and you begin to think and feel like an invalid. If you exercise too much, your muscles and joints may become inflamed. You may become over-tired so that your body doesn't have a chance to live up to your new demands and establish health. A good blend of the two, rest and exercise, will gradually improve your health and mobility. This blend is different for each person.

Some signs of 'overdoing it' are: swelling that either increases or appears where there wasn't any before you exercised; pain which doesn't go away within two or three hours after exercise; real fatigue as you do the exercises; and breathlessness during and after exercise. If you show any of these signs, slow down! You'll get better more quickly – and for longer – if you build up your level of exercise gradually.

'Underdoing it' means that you lose strength, suppleness, mobility and energy. You begin to feel stuck in the chair and to treat yourself like an invalid. Don't do it! Your general health will become poor and you may even become depressed. Try instead to improve and extend your life through exercise and interesting activities.

If you take drugs on a regular basis, ask your GP how they will affect you when you exercise. He or she may help you choose the form of exercise which will do you the most good without any worry. Aim for exercise that does not injure you in any way, either by making you tired and irritable or by causing pain or distress in any part of your body. If you begin with very gentle, very simple exercises, you will improve – safely – through perseverance. Everyone has to start somewhere, and the greatest improvement comes from the most humble beginnings. Provided you start safely and continue safely, you will gain health from your exercise practice. If you stop being safe, you stop being healthy.

All exercise should be done twice daily – morning and evening – and it is a good idea to use more than one set of exercises. For instance, if one day you are unable to go out, use an indoor exercise option instead. And if you prefer solely indoor exercise, having an alternative set of exercises at hand will prevent you getting bored.

When you begin, get as much advice as you can from your physiotherapist, exercise teacher or doctor, but then trust yourself to work in a gentle, gradual and effective way to improve your health. While you exercise, try thinking, 'I am well. My muscles and joints are getting better every time I move.' You'll notice quick improvement from the exercises in this way *and* you'll enjoy them.

Here are some of the most beneficial forms of exercise for those who suffer a rheumatic complaint. More information can be obtained about the organizations concerned by referring to the address list in the Appendix. Exercise helps these disorders in particular:

Ankylosing spondylitis	Osteoarthritis
Fibrositis	Osteoporosis
Gout	Paget's disease
Juvenile rheumatoid arthritis	Palindromic rheumatism
Lumbago	Psychogenic rheumatism
Menopausal arthritis	Rheumatoid arthritis
Myositis	Sciatica
Neuritis	

Yoga   Yoga could as well come in amongst the Lifestyle Remedies in chapter 6, for yoga is an ancient system of attaining physical, mental and spiritual health which can alter your whole attitude and approach to life.

There are many forms of yoga but Hatha yoga is the form which focuses most closely on the body – its health, its needs and its relationship with your inner self. The exercises and postures taught in Hatha yoga are suitable for all ages, in particular those who have limited mobility, are elderly, or who have done very little exercise previously. These exercises are challenging – that is, you may always improve them – but you will gain benefit from them no matter how well you perform them at first. Stretching, balancing and simple breathing techniques are all part of this practice.

The overall physical effect of the yoga practice is an increase in your mobility, flexibility and strength with improvement in your general body function. Most rheumatic sufferers report a decrease in the pain they experience and a more positive attitude to their lives. Obviously, the two go together – it is always uplifting to be free from pain! The spiritual effects of the yoga practice are yours if you want them, although most teachers do not apply philosophical or spiritual pressure. In general, greater peace of mind and a calm control are the spiritual 'side effects' from the practice of Hatha yoga. Other forms of yoga do exist should you wish for greater emphasis to be placed on this aspect.

If you decide to attend a yoga class, please ensure that your teacher is qualified by checking with your Local Adult Education Centre and/or the organization in the Appendix, which will recommend a qualified teacher in your area.

Keep Fit and Extend

The Keep Fit Association was founded in 1956 to promote physical fitness and has worked very effectively since then, primarily with women. It adheres to strict safety guidelines by ensuring that all of its teachers are thoroughly trained according to nationally established standards.

If you are suffering one of the rheumatic diseases, you may attend a keep fit session provided you discuss the nature of your disorder with the teacher. If she does not think her class will suit your personal needs she will say so and, hopefully, recommend another teacher or type of class. It is very likely however, that she will have dealt with your type of problem previously, so you can begin your classes with confidence. You will learn movements to keep your muscles toned, your circulation and breathing at their best, and your range of mobility at its safe maximum. These benefits are in themselves preventative – they may not rid you of your rheumatism, but they will keep you active, alert and possibly prevent your disorder from getting worse.

Keep fit sessions are very social occasions and, as the exercises are performed to the accompaniment of lyrical and rhythmic music, your mood is lifted, too. The Keep Fit Association (KFA) has worked hard to bring sessions into even the most rural community, and they have succeeded. You should have no trouble in finding a safe and refreshing class local to you.

Extend began as an offshoot of the Women's League of Health and Beauty and it is intended especially for men and women aged 60 and over. Teachers of Extend must have qualified as a nurse, a physiotherapist or other medical equivalent before being accepted on the teacher-training course. This precaution ensures your complete safety as you learn the exercises and is probably why so many who attend the sessions feel that they progress in 'leaps and bounds'.

The rheumatic diseases are no strangers to Extend classes so you should not feel at all hesitant in contacting your local branch. Simply give the details of your disorder and perhaps arrange to attend your first session a little early. That way you can have a few moments to meet the teacher and discuss any questions together. You will receive a great deal of personal attention in an Extend class – which does wonders for your mood and your understanding of the purpose and importance of each exercise you learn. As with keep fit, the point of the Extend movements is to maintain mobility, strength and circulation and to improve them when possible. The result is almost always a renewed interest in life, a general improvement in health, and a reduction in the pain and stiffness associated with rheumatic disorders.

Stretching and Mobility Exercises

Performing exercises which stretch your muscles and increase the mobility of your joints will reduce pain and stiffness, enhance your mood and leave you with more energy than you had before exercising. These benefits are felt especially if you exercise once in the morning and once before you go to bed. The period of exercise need be of only 10–15 minutes duration and you may be either standing or seated. No weights are used and these exercises are not intended to challenge your stamina, i.e. you should not feel breathless or fatigued.

The procedure is very simple: begin with your feet and, progressing up your body, move the main joints as far as possible without pain. This approach will improve mobility and, by the way, include some stretching. Try the sample programme on pages 82–4 for yourself.

As your suppleness and mobility improve you may wish to extend the movements you perform: if you feel you can, then do. The golden rule is to avoid pain while, at the same time, moving to the limits of your range of motion. And, of course, do the exercises twice daily.

Swimming

If you are fortunate enough to have a pool at your disposal, do take advantage of this marvellous form of exercise. Swimming invigorates by challenging your stamina and your circulation. The whole body is used in swimming and, because the water supports your body weight, you may exercise joints and muscles that are made painful or uncomfortable by other forms of exercise.

There are many popular classes held in pools specifically for this reason and you can usually find one which is either single sex or specially for your age group. The exercises performed in these classes do not necessarily require that you know how to swim. In fact, they are often held in shallow pools and you perform some of the exercises

1) Sit tall and point your toes, then pull them back towards your leg.

2) Try twisting your feet from side to side.

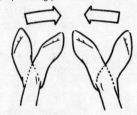

3) Circle your feet slowly once in each direction.

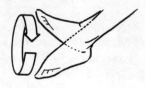

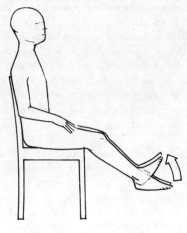

4) Sit tall and hug one knee as close to your body as you can. Hold this position for the count of five.

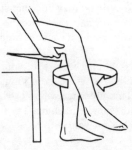

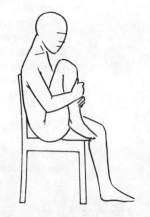

5) Lower your knee with both hands clasped under your thigh. Hold your leg slightly lifted while you circle your lower leg gently clockwise, then counter-clockwise. This movement is felt in the knee. Repeat movements 4 and 5 with the other leg.

6) Lie on your back and allow your feet to rest 'open', out to your sides. Now rotate one leg so that your foot points inward for the count of five. Repeat this movement six times with each leg, or move both legs at once. Adjust the amount of movement in each leg in order to avoid pain.

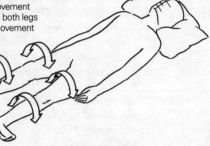

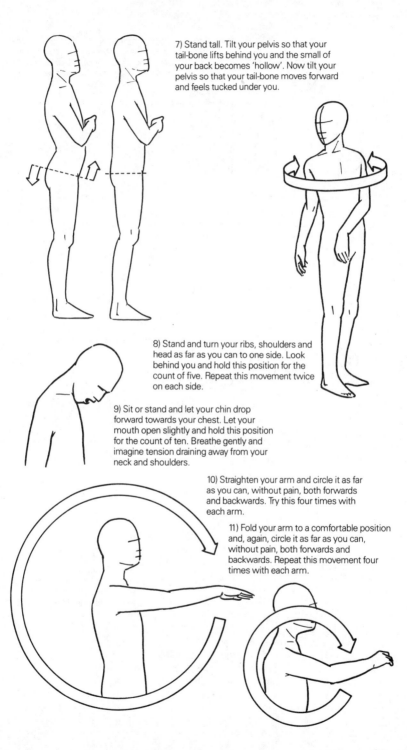

7) Stand tall. Tilt your pelvis so that your tail-bone lifts behind you and the small of your back becomes 'hollow'. Now tilt your pelvis so that your tail-bone moves forward and feels tucked under you.

8) Stand and turn your ribs, shoulders and head as far as you can to one side. Look behind you and hold this position for the count of five. Repeat this movement twice on each side.

9) Sit or stand and let your chin drop forward towards your chest. Let your mouth open slightly and hold this position for the count of ten. Breathe gently and imagine tension draining away from your neck and shoulders.

10) Straighten your arm and circle it as far as you can, without pain, both forwards and backwards. Try this four times with each arm.

11) Fold your arm to a comfortable position and, again, circle it as far as you can, without pain, both forwards and backwards. Repeat this movement four times with each arm.

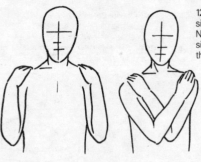

12) Touch your shoulders using their same-side hands and hold for the count of five. Now cross your hands to their opposite-side shoulders and hold this position for the count of five also.

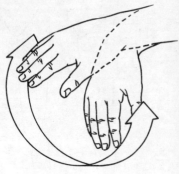

13) Relax your arms and shoulders and shake your hands loosely — as though trying to shake water from them.

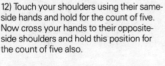

14) Open your hands, spread your fingers as far as possible and hold them stretched for the count of five. Now make fists and hold them tightly for the count of five. Repeat this movement frequently during the day.

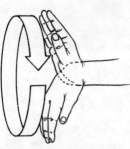

15) Let your hands relax and circle them so that your wrist rotates. Repeat this movement clockwise and counter-clockwise with each hand.

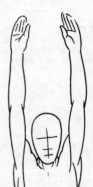

16) Stand, sit or lie on your back and breathe in as you stretch your arms up over your head as far as you can. Hold this stretch for the count of five.

17) Breathe out as you relax from the stretch and bring your elbows down towards your body. When you are ready, repeat movements 16 and 17 three more times.

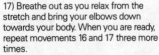

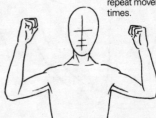

18) Hold on to the edge of the pool and tuck your legs up towards your chest. Now push your legs back and allow your body to straighten behind you. Repeat this movement slowly, three more times.

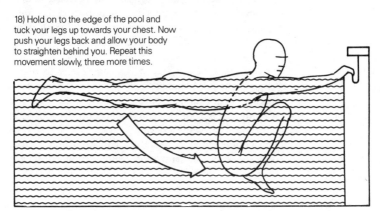

19) Stand, keeping the leg nearest the side of the pool straight. Stretch your other leg behind you, then forward...

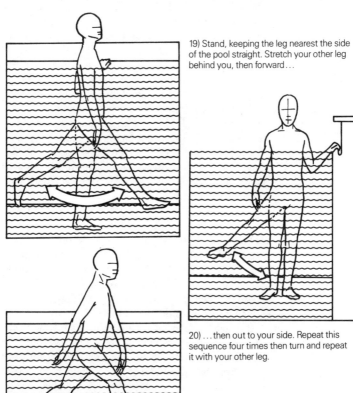

20) ...then out to your side. Repeat this sequence four times then turn and repeat it with your other leg.

21) Using the shallow end of the pool, take large 'marching' steps through the water. Hold on to the side of the pool if you like.

85

holding on to the side of the pool. Just three or four simple exercises done in water begin to mobilize the large joints and strengthen the muscles of your back, abdomen, arms and legs. Try the examples on page 85 for yourself.

If you know how to swim you may prefer to bypass the edge-of-the-pool exercises, in which case, begin by swimming a length or two using your favourite stroke. Increase the number of lengths you swim gradually and include a variety of strokes if you can.

Swimming may be practised daily or just once each week but, however frequently you swim, combine it with a daily stretching routine to keep your muscles elastic.

Walking   This is one exercise which should never be underrated. It is effective, challenging, uplifting and pleasant. Walking uses the main joints and muscles of your body and, at the same time, exercises your heart and lungs so that your circulation, muscle-tone, stamina, posture and mobility are all improved. If you walk briskly, swinging your arms at the same time, then the muscles and joints of your upper body are also exercised, while a walk uphill builds additional strength in your abdomen, thighs and lower back muscles.

Slow walking is also effective exercise and is appropriate if you have lost some mobility in your back, hips and legs. For you, a walk to and from the shops may be very slow and challenging. It is worth persevering, however. Circulation of blood and lymph is improved with gentle walking, improving the health of your joints – especially the weight-bearing joints of the lower back, hips, knees and ankles.

Your body responds to the challenge of walking by reducing levels of fat, utilizing the vitamins and minerals presented in your diet and stored in your body, and by strengthening your heart and lungs. If you pay attention to your posture while you walk, keeping as straight and tall as possible, then your mood is also improved – you feel younger, happier and more alive.

If you suffer degeneration of the hip joints, your doctor may recommend that you avoid walking, or do very little of it. In that case, once each day go 'jarmming', which is jogging with your arms! Sit tall, on the edge of a chair, and run with your arms – just like children do when they are pretending they are a steam engine. Jarmming has the benefits of walking without placing stress on your weight-bearing joints.

Whenever you walk, do your best to avoid limping as this puts extra strain on all of your other joints and eventually compounds your problem. The use of a walking stick may prevent you from limping too much.

Air and Sunlight Therapy

At the turn of the century, there was a great trend towards enjoying the benefits of clean air and sunlight. You may have seen those old, rather humorous photographs of men and women purposefully filling their lungs with sea air while baring their limbs to the sun. Well, the fashions may change, but the benefits of air and sun are real.

Air will not specifically help your rheumatic condition, but it will help *you* – your mood, your resolve to be well, your outlook on life and your general level of vitality. Cool air, breathed deeply into the lungs, stimulates the circulation and benefits your lungs and heart. Of course, you take in air every time you breathe, but air as part of a therapy should be clean, cool and from the great outdoors. Unfortunately, that may not be easy for everyone – air is often dirty or it may be difficult for you to go outdoors. But if you have a garden, patio or balcony try to use it daily, or just open your window and stand by it while you do some basic stretches. Take slow, deep breaths and, with each breath out, imagine you are breathing pain and disease out of your body.

Sunlight helps to provide some of the vitamin D your body needs by reacting with a substance in your skin called dehydrocholesterol. Vitamin D determines how well your body uses calcium and phosphorus, which are essential to the production and maintenance of healthy bone. You don't need to go nut-brown in order for sunlight to benefit you. A little bit each day – even if it's a grey day – gives you an adequate 'dose'. In fact, it is becoming more and more obvious that too much exposure to sun can contribute to the development of skin cancer. As we increasingly pollute our atmosphere, more of the sun's harmful rays get through to us and damage is more easily done to the skin.

The best, most pleasant, formula for getting air and sunlight in healthy, beneficial doses is to be outdoors doing something for about 30 minutes each day – or longer. (If you are worried about skin damage, wear a hat and a lightweight shirt with sleeves.) The more active you are during this period, the greater the benefits to your health. Walking to and from the shops, gardening, sitting in the park, feeding the birds, all of these are therapeutic – and not just for your body. You will probably sleep better at night, wake less stiff and sluggish the next day and generally feel brighter. Being outdoors helps to put pain, discomfort, worry, and depression in a better perspective.

6

'HANDS ON'

REMEDIES

The 'hands on' remedies generally consist of another person moving the joints and muscles of your body while you remain passive. It is best if this person is a qualified practitioner, although there are some occasions when you may work on your own body or when a friend or spouse may provide some basic assistance. 'Hands on' remedies require that the practitioner be sensitive to your body and mood, and knowledgeable of your illness. When this sensitivity is maintained, the 'hands on' remedies are pleasant experiences. All of the approaches described below seek to avoid pain, though if your disorder is well established or already quite painful, you may experience a small amount of pain temporarily.

In general, these treatments improve circulation of both blood and lymph, improve skin and muscle tone and increase mobility in the affected joints. However, the use of these remedies will vary according to the variety of rheumatic complaint you suffer. Inflammation is not always compatible with massage, nor osteoarthritis with joint manipulation. Your practitioner will perform what is appropriate to your needs on each respective visit. You may be surprised at what can be done. For instance, your passive involvement (you are usually reclining) often allows even stiff or painful areas to be mobilized, massaged or exercised, because the tension which would be present if those areas were taking weight or doing the work themselves is absent.

When you go for treatment, you should expect to remove some of your clothing so that you are able to move freely and give the practitioner access to the joints and muscles to be treated. Try to stay relaxed! This will get easier once you know what to expect, though relaxation established early on will make the treatment you receive more immediately effective. Refer to the Appendix at the end of this book for names and addresses of parent organizations.

Here are some of the disorders the 'hands on' remedies may help:

Ankylosing Spondylitis	Osteoarthritis
Ankylosis	Sciatica
Fibrositis	Spondylitis
Lumbago	Synovitis
Myositis	Tendinitis
Neuritis	Tenosynovitis

Osteopathy   In the mid-19th century Dr Andrew Taylor Still founded osteopathy as an alternative to what he saw as brutal and intrusive systems of medicine practised at that time. He felt strongly that the body had within it the means of healing itself, without intervention, but he also observed that if the circulation of blood was impaired in any way, illness would result. Dr Still became convinced that, provided the body's skeleton was able to move in a mechanically correct way, no impairment of circulation would occur and health would result. He observed that an ill person moved in ways which indicated an incorrect placement of the skeleton and this prevented correct functioning of the whole body. Dr Still devised osteopathy as a means of correcting misplacement in the joints of the body and practised it with great success on a great variety of ailments.

Modern osteopathy uses methods of treatment and diagnosis which are recognized and accepted within orthodox medical practice. The osteopath begins treatment by palpating, or massaging, the deep tissues of your body. These tissues are called the fascia; they are fibrous sheaths which envelop muscles, ligaments, tendons and major organs. Often this palpation is sufficient to relieve symptoms because it corrects the inhibited circulation of blood.

If further treatment is necessary, the osteopath manipulates the joints in order to free them from a rigid or incorrect position. Most often, joint misplacement is not severe, as in a dislocation. Rather, it is a position within what is called 'the normal range of movement' for that joint, but at the extremes of that range. There is usually a degree of rigidity. Any joint misplacement or rigidity inhibits circulation of the blood and, in rare cases, may even trap a nerve. Therefore the osteopath sees even minor misplacement of a joint worthy of treatment.

There are many reasons why joint misplacement may occur – injury, poor posture, pain, or stress. As part of the treatment, an osteopath will help you to re-educate your body to avoid misuse in any of these areas. So, for instance, you may be shown a series of simple exercises to perform daily at home. You may be introduced to a pleasant means of reducing your level of stress, and you will undoubtedly be shown how poor posture and poor ways of moving affect the amount of pain or discomfort you feel. These are essential aspects of osteopathy which will, if you follow them, maintain health and increase your own awareness and control of your body's function.

There are approximately 150 different manoeuvres used by an osteopath to release misplacement of the skeleton. You will experience very few of these for your particular problem, possibly as few as three or four. You may, however, be asked to make several return visits to the osteopath over the course of many months in order to maintain the corrected position and use of your body. If you perform at home the movements and exercises recommended, your muscles and connective tissues will learn to support the corrections made, your circulation will be left unimpaired and your health will improve.

Manipulation This is the practice of moving the joints of the body to correct any misplacement of them. The manner in which it is done, and the intention with which manipulation is practised, varies between osteopathy, chiropractic, physiotherapy and other manipulative practices such as kinesiotherapy. Some practitioners believe that a cure follows immediately as a result of 'freeing' a joint while others, such as osteopaths, believe that a misplaced joint can be both the result and the cause of illness and that cure is only possible over a longer period of time.

All practitioners of manipulation should avoid causing you pain. Although some pain may be felt briefly if your disorder is well established, do not accept that prolonged or severe pain is a necessary part of manipulation.

Massage Massage is an ancient practice which has always been held in high esteem for its health-giving effects. Of course, there are many approaches to massage but those of most benefit to the arthritic or rheumatic person do not cause pain. Rather, massage should be gently stimulating and invigorating. It improves your circulation, loosens the joints, releases tension from your muscles and connective tissues and tones both skin and nerves. And as a bonus, it lifts your spirits.

If your spouse or a friend massages you, it is important that they respond to your body signals with sensitivity. A trained masseur (male) or masseuse (female) will want to know about your disorder before beginning the treatment so that they may be effective and avoid causing you discomfort. They may use a little talcum powder or light oil to enable their hands to pass more smoothly over your skin. Some even combine aromatherapy (see chapter 8) with their practice of massage to heighten the effects of their treatment.

Massage, in some form, is part of many other treatments such as osteopathy and it is, in fact, the parent of physiotherapy. Most forms of rheumatic diseases benefit from massage. However, inflamed areas should not be massaged.

Physiotherapy Physiotherapy began its official life in Britain as the Chartered Society of Massage and Medical Gymnastics, founded in 1920. Later, in 1943, it became the Chartered Society of Physiotherapy which continues to this day. This practice uses manipulation, massage and exercise to adjust the structure (skeleton) of your body so that the joints, muscles, tendons, ligaments and nerves function correctly. It is therefore related to all of the previously described practices.

Although physiotherapy is usually done *to* you, while you remain quite passive, there are exercises that you may be asked to perform at home in order to maintain the improvement you have gained by visiting a qualified practitioner. A physiotherapist will use water, heat, electricity and weights as well as his or her own hands to assist you in movements or exercises that will correct your body function. Most of the rheumatic diseases can benefit from this treatment.

Physiotherapy is also used by very healthy people – such as athletes – to maintain health and prevent minor disorders from becoming major. You may visit a physiotherapist on the National Health with a recommendation from your doctor, or you may attend privately. Members of the Chartered Society of Physiotherapy are not allowed to advertise, although they are listed in the Yellow Pages.

Chiropractic   Daniel Palmer, an American, founded this science in 1895 and developed it through research and application over many years. It is based on massage and manipulation and, though it has changed since 1895 as new understanding of the body has come to light, chiropractic still adheres to the fundamental guidelines which Palmer set out.

First, Palmer observed that the correct and healthy functioning of the nerves resulted in good health, and vice versa – that good health meant healthy nerve function.

Second, he deduced that pressure applied to the nerves undermines health. This pressure could be brought about by toxins in the body, by tension in the muscles and by joints out of proper alignment.

Palmer used massage of the muscles and manipulation of the joints – especially the spine – to correct what he could of the resulting dysfunction. But he also recognized and advocated the importance of a vitamin and mineral-rich diet and plenty of exercise and fresh air to support good health and maintain any corrections which chiropractic may have incurred.

Chiropractic makes use of X-rays, urine tests and blood pressure as part of its diagnostic procedure. It considers that the techniques employed in chiropractic deal with the cause of ill-health, not just the symptoms. Of the rheumatic disorders, chiropractic has recognized success in treating sciatica, bursitis, myositis, lumbago, some forms of arthritis and many of the disorders which accompany these rheumatic complaints.

Much of the manipulation involved in treatment from a chiropractor is focused on the spine. This is because the spine is a nerve centre, with most of the nerves from the torso and extremities running into the spinal cord, and is also the most complex and vulnerable structure of the human skeleton.

Lifestyle Remedies

You may have noticed that people who live a healthy lifestyle often have a real exuberance for life. You could be one of them. When you adhere to a style of living which places wellbeing high on your list of priorities, you can look forward to a life enhanced by good health. You can develop a positive outlook which lets you enjoy your life more than ever, and you can gradually undo the habits and health problems which undermine the quality of your life.

These remedies deal with many aspects of your life, not just the symptoms of illness. They attempt to establish total health by considering each aspect of your life and how it contributes to your disorder. And they place great emphasis on your own ability to improve your present level of health and to prevent illness in the future. Each of these remedies teaches you the first steps in reclaiming that ability.

It may take you a little time to re-shape your lifestyle but this process is normally very pleasant and sometimes even exciting because the benefits you'll feel are usually fairly immediate. Most rheumatic conditions show rapid improvement when lifestyle changes such as these are begun, in particular:

Ankylosing Spondylitis	Myositis
Ankylosis	Osteoarthritis
Fibrositis	Paget's Disease
Gout	Palindromic Rheumatism
Lumbago	Psychogenic Rheumatism
Menopausal Arthritis	Rheumatoid Arthritis

Naturopathy

Naturopathy advocates that you rely on the healing power of nature to deal with illness and establish health. Nature, in this sense, includes your food, drink, movements, thoughts, hygiene, sleep and your body. Naturopaths believe that your body is qualified to heal itself and that it will always do so provided you fulfil its basic needs using only natural substances and practices.

For instance, in the naturopathic lifestyle, food should be unprocessed and organically grown when possible (a close neighbour to the raw food diet in chapter 4). Any cooking must be simply done and use little fat. Drink includes only clear fluids, avoiding coffee, tea and alcohol. Experienced naturopaths may even fast for one day each month to release toxins from the body. Regular warm or cold, but never hot, baths are taken frequently, followed by massage (if you're lucky!). Outdoor exercise is taken daily with emphasis placed on deep breathing and exposure to the sun. Some who live this lifestyle endorse nude sun-bathing in moderation. This very ancient practice makes sense even in orthodox terms because the sun's rays react with a substance in your skin, dehydrocholesterol, to make vitamin D which acts beneficially on your bones and joints.

No drugs are taken in the naturopath lifestyle unless they are part of the diet (i.e. herbs) or unless they are necessary in an emergency. Indeed, most of the over-the-counter drugs which many people take daily, such as laxatives and sleeping tablets, are unnecessary once these natural guidelines are adopted.

Naturopathy has a surprising attitude to any illness which might occur in spite of so much healthy living. It purports that illness is created by the body in an attempt to restore health and that your body becomes 'activated' by illness into a better way of life. Therefore, when a person becomes ill, the naturopath would encourage them to allow the illness to 'run its course' so that the body can be rid of it and then manifest its underlying health and strength. This belief needs you to trust your body to do what is best for you. It also needs you to accept responsibility for the lifestyle changes which might be necessary to ensure that illness does not repeat. Naturopathy works for thousands and thousands of people, many of whom happen upon the lifestyle as a last resort, when all else fails to make them healthier.

People who have practised this lifestyle for a long time are amongst the healthiest people on earth. There are various cultures around the world which live this way without ever hearing the term 'naturopathy'. They tend to live long, healthy and happy lives without the chronic ill health which plagues 'over-processed' cultures.

Naturopathy is a complete remedy. If you wish to get the feel of it (without committing yourself to the title), try combining the raw food diet (chapter 4), air and sunlight remedy (chapter 5), massage (chapter 6), positive thinking (chapter 6), and hot and cold remedies (chapter 10).

Stress Reduction

Stress is part of a normal life and even the most primitive peoples have to deal with it. Stress is real – it has physical, mental and emotional effects which can feel either beneficial and exciting or negative and worrying. Some people claim to thrive on stress, but for others it is a source of illness and anxiety. If you find stress a problem, take heart; it is probably impossible to eliminate stress from your life but it *is* possible to reduce it and to manage it so that your health is not undermined.

First, acknowledge the source of stress in your own life and observe how it develops and resolves. A visit to your GP may cause you to feel very stressful, so might receiving the gas bill. You might worry about your children, a social event, your future or something altogether less tangible. And if several such events happen in one day, your level of stress may rocket so that you feel nervous all day or have trouble sleeping. Try to pin-point the source of your stress – whether physical, mental or emotional – then notice how it acts upon your body.

It is correct for your body to change when it is undergoing any form of stress. Your hormone production, blood sugar level, rate of breathing, heart rate, digestion and level of muscular tension alter in an attempt to deal with stress. In short, you function differently. But if you 'bottle up' your stress and 'put' it in one particular area of the body, you may function incorrectly even after the stressful event has passed. Putting stress in your stomach may induce indigestion or even ulcer, while in your spine it will cause lower backache or bad posture. Dumping stress on your neck and shoulders will lead to stiffness, pain and headache. These are forms of stress management, but they are not at all beneficial. In fact, they tend to undermine your health and prevent you from getting the most from life. These habits encourage a long-term 'stacking up' of stressful symptoms that ultimately rob you of health.

To reduce the level of stress you live with, allow it to race through your body, creating the natural changes, *but then push it out*. Once you have experienced stress, get rid of it. Don't allow it to loiter about making your life miserable and unhealthy.

There are many ways of getting rid of stress. Some people go for a walk, some play a game of solitaire, feed the birds, or play with a baby; some do deep breathing, close their eyes for ten minutes, or sit in a rocking chair and stare out of the window. Others, if they are still in the stressful situation (at work, for instance), develop techniques which don't require them to stop what they are doing. These can be as diverse as making doodles while speaking on the phone to rotating their ankles while in the middle of a difficult meeting.

However, there is another aspect of stress which often goes unmentioned, even though it has particular relevance to those suffering from rheumatic disorders. That is, stress which is caused by diet, drugs and the day-to-day way you treat your body.

A diet high in sugar, salt, fats and processed foods creates a great deal of stress for your body. All of your body's systems – circulation, digestion, elimination, and so on – have to work very much harder when you consume these foods regularly or in quantity. And they don't like to work hard because hard work causes stress – it means an uncomfortable change in the way your systems function. Very soon, complications develop which can lead to disease.

Similarly, with drugs, no matter how they ease the symptoms of a disease, your body still has to work very hard to put them through its systems. Again, this is stressful and you will notice that, often, additional disease is *created* through use of drugs.

Normally, when dealing with stress, you can allow your body its reaction and then remove yourself from the stressful influence. But if you are continually taking foods or drugs that create *more* stress, then your body has no chance to recover from the changes it naturally goes through to manage stress. The prognosis is poor, then, because your body spirals out of control – you lose a sense of what is stressful and what isn't and come to live in a virtually permanent state of tension.

Arthritis and rheumatism can be stress-related diseases. Some forms are due to emotional trauma which alters the hormonal balance in the body, causing it to function in a state of stress. Some are initiated by injury which creates stressful function in one particular region, while others seem to be the result of long-term misuse of the body, for example through drugs and bad diet, causing stress which ultimately develops into disease.

Here are the steps you can take to reduce stress in your life:

● Understand that stress has physical effects, no matter what its source.

● Allow yourself to feel stressful when necessary, but don't let the feeling linger.

● Adopt a healthy diet – low in salt, sugar, meat, fat and processed foods.

● Minimize the number of drugs you take.

● Try including an anti-stress activity in your daily life, such as a sport or game, a form of meditation, a walk or a special time set aside to read a book or listen to music.

There are many formalized types of stress management, too, and some addresses for your reference are given in the Appendix.

Relaxation Techniques and Biofeedback

'Relax!' It is easy to say and easy to imagine but, for many people, difficult to do. Perhaps if you learn what relaxation is and how it is beneficial you may find it easier to achieve. Here is an experiment for you to try: make a strong fist to show off your bicep (however diminutive) by clenching your fist and forearm. This is tension. Now undo your fist and slacken your bulging bicep. This is relaxation.

It is *nearly* as simple as that. What you have just experienced is muscular tension and muscular relaxation which, if done regularly with all the major muscles, can create mental and emotional relaxation as well. One relaxation technique in particular teaches a tense/relax sequence to help you reduce stress, revitalize your body and establish better posture and use of muscle. Try this simple sequence:

● Lie flat on the floor with your arms a little distance from your sides and your feet about 12 inches (30 cm) apart
● To begin, tense your lower body by curling your toes, tightening your calf muscles, then your thigh muscles and then clenching your buttocks
● Hold this tension for the count of five
● Then let the tension go – let your legs feel very heavy
● Next, tense your upper body by bringing your chin close to your neck
● Make fists of your hands and tighten the muscles in your forearms
● Tighten the muscles in your upper arms and shoulders
● Breathe out and tighten your abdomen muscles
● Hold this tension for the count of five
● Then let the tension go – let your breath become deep and roll your head from side to side. Let your shoulders and arms feel heavy
● Finally, tense both your lower and upper body together. You may do this one step at a time, as listed above, or all at once so that your muscles become tense simultaneously. Hold your whole body tense for the count of five and then let the tension go.
● You may repeat this process two or three times.

Taking yourself through this tense/relax cycle gives you greater awareness of what your muscles are doing. Once you have this awareness, you will find it easier to control the degree of tension you allow in yourself.

Muscular relaxation benefits many arthritic disorders because it can reduce pain. Pain that is caused by the ends of bone grating together is unlikely to be reduced by relaxing muscles, but pain which accompanies other rheumatic conditions, or that is due to muscle spasm, can be minimized by relaxing the muscles around the afflicted joint.

Biofeedback uses a machine which allows you to see or hear biological information from your body that you might not otherwise receive. This is done by attaching electrode pads to your fingers, palms, feet or face. The electrodes measure your skin temperature, your blood pressure, your brain-wave patterns or other of your body functions. This information is then presented to you – through the machine – as a sound or a visual image.

It is possible for you, by receiving this 'new' information, to learn to control pain, migraine headaches, sleeplessness, backaches and a variety of other physical or mental states after just a few biofeedback sessions. If this technique appeals to you, it is worth asking your doctor or natural medicine practitioner about the availability of biofeedback training in your area. Although the machines are initially quite expensive, some biofeedback groups have made a joint purchase of the equipment which is then shared on a rota, or library basis.

Other relaxation methods focus more on your mental and emotional state. Indeed, you may have noticed that muscle relaxation or biofeedback improved your mood and general outlook. Use of concentration, breathing patterns or sound can help you to achieve a state of calm, unconscious relaxation in body, mind and spirit.

| Positive Thinking | Thinking positive thoughts creates energy. People throughout history have shown how hope and belief can change lives – from illness, despair and poverty many have created health, happiness and success for themselves by deciding that they can. |

For you, suffering from a rheumatic disorder, deciding to be positive in your thoughts and actions may be the very first step on your way to improving your health. Here are some positive guidelines:

● Make a decision to be as positive as you can, all the time.

● Now, face up to the facts of your disorder – what is it, how long will it be with you, what do you think caused it?

● Become responsible for your disorder. In other words, do as much as *you* can to ease it or remedy it rather than relying solely on others.

● Begin to undermine your disorder by refusing to allow it to control your life.

● Look beyond your pain and discomfort to the activities and achievements you still desire – and do your utmost to accomplish them!

● Adopt practical changes in your life, from the many

suggestions in this book, that will help you to give your positive attitude real effect.

Positive thinking is a powerful medicine within each of us, just waiting to be accepted into our lives.

Mind Cure and Visualization

Mind cure has existed in various forms throughout history with more or less emphasis placed on its religious, or divine, aspect. The Chinese called their version The Happiness Cure, more recent versions are Christian Science and Joy Philosophy. Mind cure is based on a belief in a divine element within all life. It purports that to inspire health you must think 'good' thoughts – loving, caring, hopeful, courageous, kind and healthy – which allow divinity to live within you. To become ill, you need only think 'bad' thoughts that block the divine element from your life.

The mind cure philosophy states that if you live your life welcoming all that is presented to you, illness may be prevented and overcome. For those who already suffer, mind cure teaches that 'right thinking' will remedy the disease. Summarized in popular terms – you are what you think.

The effects of mind cure on rheumatic disorders are similar to those from positive thinking, stress reduction and relaxation. Through your own attitudes and determination you may gradually begin to surface from the pain, despair and illness which prevent your health improving as it could.

There is a further, more active step you can take towards treating your disorder with your mental powers. It is called **visualization** and it is a method of directing and controlling your body's inbuilt healing powers towards your affliction. In this method, you concentrate fully on a mental picture of, for instance, your arthritic hip joint. Once you have secured this picture in your mind, imagine the circulation of healthy blood all around this joint. Imagine next a battle fought, in your hip, between health and illness. Then imagine the defeat of illness and the conquering glow of health in your hip. Resume your normal activities, but repeat the visualization later in the day and continue daily until you feel a definite improvement in your disorder.

This is just one example of the power of visualization. There are many specific techniques and thought patterns which you may learn in order to improve your control of illness. Alternatively, you can easily devise your own internal images once you gain confidence in the ability of your mind to create health. See the Appendix for further reading.

Homoeopathy and biochemics are natural healing methods which focus on building health rather than combating illness. Both consider the symptoms of illness to be your body's natural and correct response to disease. Therefore, in both forms of treatment, symptoms are not suppressed but are stimulated so that the underlying disease may be overcome by your body's own natural efforts.

Medicines from both systems actively support and enhance your body's natural response to illness. All homoeopathic and biochemic medicines are completely safe, even for babies, and are entirely natural. There are no side effects from these medicines and they are not toxic in any way.

Here are some particular disorders which these remedies may help:

Bursitis	Menopausal arthritis
Dry joint	Neuritis
Fibrositis	Osteomyelitis
Gout	Osteoporosis
Infective arthritis	Sciatica
Lumbago	Tuberculous arthritis

Homoeopathic Remedies

The principle behind the homoeopathic approach to healing is very old and has been described frequently in simple terms such as 'like cures like', 'fight fire with fire', 'the hair of the dog', and so on. In practice, this principle means that substances which create symptoms of disease in a healthy person can, in smaller doses, establish health in a sick person suffering those same symptoms. This system was formalized by Dr Samuel Hahnemann in the early 19th century and has been in use as homoeopathy ever since.

Hahnemann is often quoted as saying, 'Treat the patient, not the disease', and this has become the focus of homoeopathic prescribing. For example, if you and your neighbour went to your GP and were both diagnosed as having rheumatoid arthritis you might both expect to receive the same medical prescription. If you both then decided to visit a homoeopathic doctor, you and your neighbour would probably come away from this visit with different remedies for the same disease! This is because the homoeopath was treating *you* – your body, your mental state, your emotional state, your way of life – not just your disease.

Homoeopathy relies on your body's innate ability to heal itself. This means that it allows symptoms of illness to appear and does not try to suppress them. This might, at first, seem frightening, but if the symptoms are allowed to manifest while your body's underlying health is supported with homoeopathic remedies, then the disease will 'run its course'. The symptoms will disappear and you will come out of the experience more healthy than if you had suppressed the symptoms with orthodox medicine.

It is possible to treat yourself using homoeopathic remedies. However, if after four or five days of self-treatment you do not notice any improvement, you should visit a homoeopathic doctor who will give you a full interview and suggest a remedy to suit you. If you do not select the right remedy for yourself, no harm is done as all homoeopathic remedies are non-toxic. If you select the right remedy, then expect a reaction – often a temporary worsening of your symptoms. This reaction is sometimes called a 'healing crisis' and is simply a turning point in the course of your illness. It is easier to deal with this when you know what it is, but if you have a homoeopathic doctor you may wish to ring him or her at this time for a bit of support and encouragement! If your symptoms get very much worse, stop taking the remedy until the symptoms die down. Then continue taking the remedy but increase the length of time between doses. Avoid, if possible, strong foods or drinks – such as coffee, meat and alcohol – while taking homoeopathic remedies.

As you change and become more healthy, so your homoeopathy remedy may change. This is as it should be and you will notice that you gradually become more aware and 'in tune' with your body and your needs.

Here are some of the more common homoeopathic remedies for self-treatment of rheumatic disorders.

Arnica: If you suffer from gout or rheumatism and feel worse when touched, when moving, when in damp or cold environments. Your symptoms have probably come on suddenly.

Bryonia: If you suffer from rheumatic complaints which are made much worse through movement so that you prefer to lie still. You may feel irritable, often extremely so, and are at times offensive to others. You prefer to be cool rather than warm and you probably eat a lot with cravings for meat or other heavy foods. You are usually 'dry' – that is, you may have dry coughs, tend towards thirst and constipation and feel your pain as sharp or stabbing. This remedy is most effective when your disease is at its worst or nearly so.

Calcarea Fluorica (Calc. Fluor.): This remedy is recommended in gout with swellings in the finger joints and in lumbago with a very deep sensation of pain. Warm conditions usually make you feel better and you find that once you are moving the pain is eased somewhat. You may tend to have catarrh.

Rhus Toxicodendron (Rhus tox.): Many of the rheumatic disorders are improved with the use of this remedy, in particular lumbago, sciatica and aches in the joints and surrounding tissue. You feel a restless urge to move and, even though this is painful to start with, your condition improves with movement. Your discomfort worsens at night when you may also feel anxious and somewhat fearful. Cold and damp conditions make you feel worse and you even tend to avoid cold drinks. You may suffer from diarrhoea and skin complaints. This remedy is most effective when your condition is at its worst or nearly so.

Homoeopathic remedies are taken in granule (also called pilule) or tincture form. Granules are tiny tablets which are dissolved on the tongue. Tinctures are alcohol-based solutions which you further dilute in water.

One dose in granule form = 1 or 2 granules (tablets). In acute conditions take one dose every two hours for twelve hours (six doses). Following that, or in less acute cases, take one dose between each meal (three times each day) until the condition improves. You may then reduce the number of doses you take each day, or stop taking the remedy altogether.

When using a homoeopathic tincture, dilute five drops of it in a small glass of water and take sips from this glass throughout the day. Prepare a fresh dilution each day. Store the *unmixed* tincture in a cool, dark place – it will keep indefinitely. This method is slightly less portable than the granules and is therefore best for home use.

To begin your treatment, use the homoeopathic remedies labelled 6th potency. For an acute condition you may use the 30th potency over a period of three or four days. However, you may wish to consult a homoeopathic doctor or chemist to confirm your need for this strength remedy.

Biochemic Tissue Salts

Dr Wilhelm H. Schuessler established, in the early part of this century, that the human body is composed of twelve basic mineral salts and that a deficiency in one or more of them results in illness. These salts are inorganic, but are present in living tissue as essential elements of health. Schuessler developed a means of presenting these salts to the body in minute homoeopathic doses which are readily assimilated into the blood and therefore quickly circulated through the body.

Biochemic tissue salts are produced as tablets which dissolve quickly on the tongue. An adult dose is four tablets, a child's dose is two, and an infant's dose is one tablet. The size of the dose does not increase the effect of the tissue salt, but the frequency with which you take the dose does. So, for instance, in chronic conditions you should take one dose between each meal (three times each day). For acute conditions, take one dose every half hour until relief is apparent, at which time begin to increase the length of time between doses. Tissue salts, like homoeopathic remedies, are entirely harmless and will not cause adverse side effects.

Schuessler developed twelve tissue salts as the foundation of biochemics. These twelve are all that are essential in order to maintain health and are packaged with their homoeopathic abbreviation as well as their number (e.g. Ferr. Phos.; Tissue salt 4). Later, however, eighteen combinations of tissue salts were devised and they are packaged with the homoeopathic abbreviations of their salts and a letter (e.g. Mag. Phos., Nat. Mur., Silica; Combination H). Latterly, six additional remedies have been developed for specific conditions bringing the total number of tissue salt preparations available to thirty-six. The following are those recommended for rheumatic conditions.

Calc. Fluor. (Calcium Fluoride): For rheumatic conditions where the joints are enlarged and in lumbago accompanied by a strained and dragging sensation. Use this remedy in diseases which affect the bone surface.

Calc. Phos. (Calcium Phosphate): Associated with nutrition and the formation of bone. Use this tissue salt in cases of rickets, lumbago and osteoporosis. Poor circulation, numbness and a feeling of cold are often accompanying disorders.

Ferr. Phos. (Iron Phosphate): The tissue salt which improves the oxygen-carrying ability of the blood. For this reason, pain and inflammation of all sorts are relieved when Ferr. Phos. is taken. In particular, strained muscles, stiff neck, lumbago and other rheumatic afflictions of the back, swollen finger joints and rheumatic conditions made worse through movement are eased by taking this remedy.

Kali. Mur. (Potassium Chloride): When your rheumatic condition comes on suddenly and includes inflammation, this tissue salt is a useful remedy. You may wish to take it alternately with Ferr. Phos.

Mag. Phos. (Magnesium Phosphate): Specifically for relieving pain. Both nerve pain, as in sciatica and neuritis, and pain caused by muscle spasm, as in back-ache, is eased when you take Mag. Phos. This tissue salt is more effective if you take a sip of warm water with the tablet.

Nat. Phos. (Sodium Phosphate): Neutralizes an acid state of your blood and prevents the deposit of acids in and around the joints. Therefore, rheumatic conditions such as gout, fibrositis and sudden attacks of rheumatism are eased when you take Nat. Phos.

Nat. Sulph. (Sodium Sulphate): Prevents the build up of fluids in the body. Therefore, gout, fibrositis and the sudden onset of rheumatism with inflammation is prevented or eased through the use of this tissue salt.

Silica (Silicic Oxide): Acts as the body's cleanser and is useful in rheumatic conditions which appear suddenly. It helps to remove toxins from the body and may be of use in rheumatic disorders where pus, swelling or infection is involved.

Combination Remedies:

Ferr. Phos., Kali Phos., Mag. Phos.: For pain, primarily non-muscular, such as that felt in sciatica and neuritis.

Calc. Fluor., Calc. Phos., Kali Phos., Nat. Mur.: For back-ache and lumbago where the joints are not adequately supported by the surrounding tissues. These conditions may be accompanied by piles.

Ferr. Phos., Kali Sulph., Mag. Phos.: For rheumatic complaints predominantly affecting the connective tissues, such as fibrositis.

Nat. Phos., Nat. Sulph., Kali Mur., Calc. Phos.: For any rheumatic condition, in particular those which include inflammation and tenderness.

To select the correct remedy, it is important that you make note of all your symptoms, even those which are mild. Then match those symptoms with the characteristics. You may find that more than one remedy is indicated. In these cases, however, one remedy will deal with the more obvious symptoms and should be taken first.

The tissue salts will keep indefinitely in their airtight containers when stored in a cool, dark cupboard. Their use will not interfere with other medicines you may be taking.

8

REMEDIES
FROM PLANTS

Plants are probably humankind's oldest and most successful form of medicine. In our diet, plants supply vitamins, minerals and other trace elements and act in a medicinal way to prevent illness. Certain plants do not constitute part of our diet yet their healing value has been recognized and put to use over the centuries to remedy chronic or acute illness. Early knowledge of the healing power of plants was probably gained by observing animals as they selected plants to cure their illnesses. Then, over thousands of years, people developed an expertise and confidence in their use of healing plants and this was passed on meticulously from generation to generation.

Plant medicine is, in some respects, the father of modern orthodox medicine yet it is currently considered an 'alternative' or 'fringe' form. This attitude is reflective of how we have lost touch, not only with our own health, but with the natural remedies which have always been available to us. Every culture on the planet has a 'pharmacy' of plants which grow within its locale and provide natural treatments for illness. But, in recent years, doubt and condemnation have undermined the use of these natural medicines and we have turned, instead, to synthetic and highly potent manufactured drugs.

The beauty of plant medicine lies in the blend of constituents present in every plant, some in such small quantities that they have been neither measured nor named. Nature has placed the 'active ingredient' of each plant in amongst these other constituents in order to modify and control its effect on the human body.

Orthodox medicine has taken its lead from plant medicine and, observing the action a healing plant has upon the body, has, in a great many cases, isolated the active ingredient and either given it alone to treat illness or made a synthetic copy of it. Here, say advocates of plant medicine, is where the dramatic and dangerous side effects of so many modern drugs are born. The modifying influence of the other constituents within the plant are crucial to the efficacy and safety of plant medicine. When removed, the 'active ingredient' is concentrated, immoderate in its action and liable to cause adverse reactions.

Orthodox medicine argues that, although side effects do occur, its method allows consistency in the measurement of both dosage and effects, while plants used naturally vary greatly in their strength and effect according to their size, where they are grown, when they are gathered, and how they are prepared. There is some truth in this argument – plants *do* vary greatly in their effect for all of these reasons. However, qualified practitioners of plant medicine are trained to consider all aspects of the plants they use before administering them as a remedy.

The discussion has gained momentum in the last decade. The following are examples of plant medicine practised in Britain. In all cases it is wise to obtain a diagnosis from your GP before considering plant remedies.

Diseases which may benefit from plant remedies are:

Bursitis	Myositis
Fibrositis	Palindromic rheumatism
Lumbago	Psychogenic rheumatism

Herbal Medicine You have, at some time, probably sipped a cup of mint or chamomile tea on the advice of a friend or neighbour that it would relieve a headache or calm your nerves. Whether or not you believed the claims made, you were using a herb as a medicine in the tradition of many generations before you. Herbalism makes use of the plant in its natural state or in a variety of prepared forms such as infusion, decoction, tablets or extract.

Self-diagnosis and then self-treatment is common but not always recommended if you wish to use plant medicine. In the event of confusing, prolonged or acute symptoms, it is wise to get a diagnosis of your problem from a doctor or a medical herbalist. Once a diagnosis is made, you may choose a herbal treatment to remedy your problem.

Here are some herbal remedies for rheumatic and arthritic complaints which you may use safely, in the suggested doses, without consulting a herbalist. Other, more powerful, herbal remedies are available, but you should first visit a qualified practitioner for guidance in their use. (See Appendix for guide to qualified practitioners.)

Comfrey: Comfrey (*Symphytum officinale*) is also called knitbone or bone-set. It has been in use for hundreds of years for its effect on healing wounds and injuries. The leaves, applied externally, reduce inflammation and encourage quick healing of damaged tissue. For internal use, comfrey is still available in the form of tablets and tea. However, *the safety of comfrey for internal use is currently being questioned and you may wish to use it as an external treatment only.* Comfrey is reputed to ease, or even eliminate, the pain and stiffness of most rheumatic disorders when used regularly. Some people grow their own comfrey and put in a few leaves as they run a bath.

Dandelion and nettle: Both of these herbs may be purchased dried for making tea. They are tonic herbs, having a cleansing effect on the blood. Both are rich in minerals, reduce acidity in the blood and, with regular use, prevent constipation. They affect the rheumatic disorders by reducing the level of toxins in the blood and thereby help to eliminate pain.

Senna and cascara: Both are natural laxatives which can be purchased in tablet or natural form. Constipation can be a major problem associated with the rheumatic diseases. Poor circulation and loss of mobility are usually the cause, although a highly-processed diet will add to the problem. Senna is a strong laxative and can, if large quantities are taken, cause stomach pains. Cascara is less powerful, though effective.

Elderflower and yarrow: A tea made from these two herbs, together, will induce perspiration and improve your circulation. Both of these actions help to reduce pain by removing the toxins from your system. Keep warm for an hour after drinking this tea.

A great many herbal preparations are available in tea, tablet or tonic form which promise to treat your rheumatism. Please contact a medical herbalist if you are unsure which would do you the most good.

Floritherapy

Have you ever wondered why the Romans wore wreaths of flowers on their heads – especially when they were feasting? The answer is that they believed in the healing power of flowers – (and that they would limit the effects of too much wine!)

Floritherapy is healing through the influence of flowers and has a long and reputable history. Generally, in season, locally grown flowers are used for their effect on the mood and on the body's natural healing powers. Flowers are selected for their colour, scent and innate characteristics to match the person and the symptoms displayed. It is believed that an 'atmosphere' conducive to healing is thus created within the person.

Modern floritherapy has established itself in the other plant remedies, in particular the Bach Flower Remedies.

Aromatherapy

Aromatherapy – the belief that aromatic substances such as flowers, fruit, spices and herbs have an effect on mood and health – has been used for thousands of years in the form of perfume, incense, pot-pourris, sachets and scented amulets. Aromatic substances – alone or in combination – have been used to disinfect, induce sleep, uplift the mood, encourage romance and dispel illness. The Bible and other histories record the use of plants in this way but, sadly, much of the unwritten expertise in aromatherapy from ancient times has been lost.

Today aromatherapy is reclaiming its place in the natural remedies medicine chest. Aromatic oils are used in combination with massage techniques as the most popular (and effective) form of aromatherapy practised specifically for health. The following is a list of aromatic oils used especially to treat rheumatic disorders:

Basil	Rosemary
Eucalyptus	Sage
Lavender	Thyme

Do not take aromatic oils internally. Instead, put a few drops in your bath or rub a small amount on to the painful place after a warm bath and wrap the area in a warm towel. See Appendix for suppliers and further reading.

Bach Flower Remedies

Dr Edward Bach began developing his flower remedies in the early part of this century after first qualifying as a medical doctor. He believed that the personality of an ill person was more important than the disease and he sought, from the very start of his medical practice, to devise a means of treating disease through the personality. In this respect his work has links with homoeopathy, although one hundred years separate Bach and Hahnemann.

Bach was a natural observer of human nature and he had often seen how an individual's mood governed an illness. While continuing his work as a medical doctor, he gradually formulated simple descriptions of the moods and behaviour which he saw over and over again in the people he was treating. He began with seven, then twelve, and finally thirty-eight different mood descriptions which he felt governed health. Bach came to see mood as the underlying cause of disease and believed that cure was possible through the removal or alteration of mood. After nearly twenty years, Bach left orthodox medical practice in order to research a means of curing disease by affecting the mood of the patient.

Bach was determined that cure should be achieved through natural, painless means. He achieved this, after years of work, by 'potentizing' flowers, which he thought of as the essence of nature, just as mood was the essence of health. His flower remedies were gradually developed in homoeopathic doses to match the thirty-eight moods he had summarized. They have been used with great success both during his lifetime and in the years since his death in 1936.

All of these remedies are harmless, no matter who takes them and in what quantity. They are free from adverse side effects and are entirely natural, both in their preparation and in their effect. The medical diagnosis of your disorder has little to do with the treatment you choose but the way you *feel* has everything to do with your selection. Therefore, your flower remedy may vary as your mood, or feelings, change.

Up to six different flower remedies may be taken at once. Select those which match your personality at the moment and add two drops from each remedy to 1 fl oz (25 ml) of spring water in a tiny bottle. This is for use within the following three weeks and should be stored in a cool, dark place. Your dose is four drops of this blend in a teaspoon of water at least four times each day, more often if you like. In particular, try to take the remedy first thing in the morning and last at night. Hold the liquid in your mouth for a few seconds before swallowing.

For acute conditions, dilute two drops each of the selected remedies in a small tumbler of water and take frequent sips over the course of the day.

Fomentations, Liniments, Ointments and Poultices

Some plants are most effective in cases of arthritis or rheumatism when applied to the body, rather than ingested. It is usual to prepare the plants in some way to increase their effectiveness.

● A **fomentation** is a strong brew made from the plant or plants you are using. The plant matter is washed, drained and usually chopped or torn before being added to water, which is then boiled. The lid is generally left off the pot and a strong simmer is maintained until the amount of liquid in the pot has diminished by half – usually about 15–20 minutes.

Allow the fomentation to cool until of a tolerable temperature, then soak a clean towel in it, wring and apply immediately to the painful or inflamed area. Put another towel in the pot ready to replace the first towel when it becomes cool. Continue for 20–30 minutes. Fomentations are employed primarily to reduce inflammation. Plants commonly used are comfrey, alder, pine needles and seaweed.

● A **liniment** is an oil or oily substance which contains the essence of the plant and is rubbed on to the affected area. You can buy liniments, use aromatic oils or make your own by soaking the plant matter in warm, clean oil – either olive or almond. Liniments are generally used to warm the painful area by increasing circulation. Make your own from chamomile, thyme, bay leaves or rosemary, or buy proprietary mixtures such as Tiger Balm or Olbas Oil.

● An **ointment** is a thick mixture of ingredients for rubbing on to the body. It contains the plant ingredient as an oil, a tincture, a powder or a water and this is mixed with a base, such as chalk or salt. Ointments are applied locally to soothe an aching or inflamed joint. Eucalyptus, thyme, rosemary and chamomile are some popular ingredients. Weleda's Rheuma Ointment is one example of a proprietary ointment.

● A **poultice** is the plant matter itself, applied to an area of pain, inflammation, heat or swelling. It imparts the healing value of the plant as well as increasing circulation to the affected area. Comfrey, mustard, alder and ginger are examples of plants used in this way. Generally, the plant matter is prepared by slight cooking, grating or mashing before being held in place with a warm towel or cloth.

9

REMEDIES
THAT YOU
WEAR

You might be lucky and own a piece of amber, or you may have to settle for an old chestnut or an EverReady battery. According to ancient and modern folklore, these items may be worn to prevent or cure the rheumatic diseases. Most folklore is hearsay, stories passed by word of mouth, and amber, chestnuts and batteries are just three of the more common items which have been credited with healing rheumatism. It is unwise to mock these claims for, undoubtedly, they have worked for someone. But as to *why* they work, we are mostly left guessing. Perhaps there is a magnetic exchange between item and wearer? Or a degree of mineral absorption through the skin? Or perhaps it is something altogether more psychological, as though the item were a talisman or amulet which helps create belief in your own health?

Here are three more items, also to be worn, which have a slightly stronger history of success. Try one if you like!

Potatoes

Some people believe that because potatoes are part of the nightshade family they poison the system and provoke rheumatic suffering when eaten. But another belief virtually contradicts this, stating instead that potatoes can provide a remedy for the rheumatic disorders when worn upon or otherwise applied to the body.

At one period in history this belief was so widespread that small pockets were sewn into clothing especially to hold potatoes. Later, raw potato juice or warm potato broth was applied to gouty or rheumatic joints. Towels soaked in the liquid were wrapped around the joint and replaced often. Sometimes slices of raw potato were placed over the painful or swollen area. This method was – and is – used for lumbago, sciatica and synovitis as well as gout and general rheumatism with claims that it relieves pain and inflammation. This remedy does not alter your constitution, therefore it is probably not a cure. Potatoes are rich in minerals and possibly some of these are absorbed through the skin.

Copper Bracelets

When Europeans first settled in Africa, they found many tribes which appeared to be entirely free from rheumatic diseases. The reason for this enviable freedom from pain appeared to be that the members of the tribes always wore at least one copper bangle. Of course, the Europeans tried it for themselves and now thousands of people all around the world swear by the beneficial effects of wearing pure copper.

Very few scientific studies have taken place to test this widespread faith in copper. Those that have been performed observe that a copper bracelet loses some of its weight over a period of time. This phenomenon has been attributed in part to your body's ability to absorb copper through the skin. But why should that matter to your rheumatism?

Well, it is likely that the copper already present in your body (yes, you do need small amounts of it) helps to remove toxins from your system which could otherwise create pain and inflammation. But many rheumatic sufferers are deficient in copper and, in those people, the job of preventing pain and inflammation isn't being done. Increasing the level of copper in the body, however, would probably reduce pain and swelling.

Knowing all of that, the obvious answer is to wear something copper against your skin. Your skin will breathe, perspire and react to the copper so that some of it may be absorbed into your system. (Note: do not wear the bracelet over an open sore or wound.) The toxins which have helped to make your life painful may be released from your body and your suffering may diminish.

Copper bracelets have worked for a great many people and there is no harm in trying one yourself. Many attractive and lightweight copper bracelets or amulets are available on the market. This is a simple, comfortable treatment suitable especially for sufferers of osteo- and rheumatoid arthritis.

Crystals

For centuries crystals have been worn to create and maintain balance and harmony in the body – specifically, to improve the health of the 'subtle' or ethereal body, that which is not apparent in X-rays or anatomical textbooks. Crystals are usually clear quartz formations, although many types of stone are worn according to personal preference.

A person who has worn a crystal for a long period of time can observe it changing as their health changes – becoming cloudy in times of imbalance and clear when harmony has been restored. Crystals are used as a focus for healing energy and this energy can be focused inward, upon the wearer, or towards another when the crystal is passed close to them. The crystal responds to the person being treated by indicating diseased areas and the degree of disharmony present. This reaction may be due to vibrations – either psychic or magnetic – given off by the person under care.

There are an increasing number of people who use crystal therapy to heal others. They use the crystal alone or with other remedies in order to create rapid and holistic health benefits.

Crystal therapy seems to cross the several boundaries between diagnostic, remedial and psychological medicine and there is much that is inexplicable and unmeasured about it. Whether or not you are attracted to or believe in the powers of crystal therapy, it seems possible that the crystal can in some way reflect the mineral content of your bones, or indeed your whole body. And, as with copper bracelets, some of the mineral content of crystals may be absorbed into your body and in that way benefit your health.

10

WATER

REMEDIES

Water has always been used, internally and externally, to improve health. The importance of water as a therapeutic substance is included in the history of virtually every culture since ancient times. It is probable that animals gave us our first indication of its healing qualities and that, by observing their use of different pools and springs, we humans were able to learn which waters healed various disorders.

Water treatments are also called hydrotherapy or hydropathy, and some have long been credited with improving the rheumatic diseases. It is these remedies which are discussed below. Water therapy may benefit the following disorders in particular:

Dry joint	Neuritis
Fibrositis	Osteoarthritis
Gout	Poncet's rheumatism
Juvenile rheumatoid arthritis	Pott's disease
Lumbago	Rheumatoid arthritis
Menopausal arthritis	Sciatica
Myositis	Spondylitis

Hot and Cold Therapy

Heat in general and hot water in particular dilates the blood vessels and enables better muscle function. In the rheumatic joint, heat often reduces pain and increases movement in the joint. Therefore, heat is useful to build the strength and mobility which can improve the rheumatic condition.

Cold water improves respiration, circulation and the mood. Apart from total body immersion, it is most effective applied to the feet, spine and hips. Sometimes cold water is used by itself to reduce inflammation. In these cases ice is packed around the afflicted area or a fine spray of very cold water is directed at the inflammation. Once the inflammation is reduced, pain and stiffness are also eased.

You can see how alternate hot and cold water baths, showers or foot baths can challenge your body's healing ability. The gradual reduction of inflammation, followed closely by improved use of muscle, creates a swift reversal in the rheumatic process. Hot and cold therapy may be applied in several ways and is included in many of the water treatments which follow.

If you are being treated at home, the best pattern to follow is a 10–15 second experience of heat, then of cold, and so on for several minutes. It is best to have someone there to help you maintain the correct temperature differences between the hot and cold. An easier method than bowls or baths of water is, for some joints, the use of hot and cold towels. These are wrapped around the afflicted joint and replaced often to maintain the correct temperatures.

Inflammation is reduced and circulation stimulated with the alternate hot and cold treatment. Repeat twice daily for one week. Have a break then and repeat the treatment if necessary.

Sitz Baths and Foot Baths

These baths are most effective when used for alternate hot and cold water therapy or with bath salts. A sitz bath is a hip bath and may be employed alone or at the same time as a foot bath. Both can control the body temperature so that pain and inflammation are reduced. Here are some examples of their use in rheumatic conditions.

● Especially for a general rheumatic feeling or for gout in its non-acute stage: take a hot foot bath (with Epsom salts) for ten minutes, keeping your upper body very warm. Now immerse your feet in a cold water bath (without salts) for five minutes while another hot foot bath is prepared. Repeat the hot and cold baths once more so that you break into a sweat. Keep very warm, dry your feet and cover them then go to bed. This remedy is excellent for improving circulation and removing toxins from your body.

● For arthritis in the hips, lumbago or sciatica: take a hot sitz bath for five minutes. Once seated, wrap a blanket to cover both your feet and your shoulders. Follow by a two-minute cold sitz bath, again wrapping the blanket around you. Repeat these two baths once again then dry yourself with a rough towel, dress in warm, loose clothes and immediately perform gentle stretches for five minutes. Try to repeat this whole sequence once again on the same day. This will improve circulation and mobility in the afflicted area.

● For a general rheumatic feeling: take a warm sitz bath and, at the same time, a cold foot bath. After five minutes, top up the sitz bath with warm water and change the foot bath to a hot one. Five minutes later, change the foot bath to a cold one and, again, top up the sitz bath. If you prefer, you may place one foot in a hot bath, the other in a cold bath and after five minutes reverse them. Throughout, keep your upper body warm – perhaps by wrapping a blanket round yourself. This treatment may cause you to perspire – another way your body flushes toxins from the blood. You will certainly notice that your circulation and mobility are improved by it.

Spas and Saunas

A spa is a form of health centre built up around a natural spring, and its water is used in a variety of ways to promote health. The water remedies described above are used in spa treatment – and more besides. Spa therapies include hot and cold baths, hot and cold showers, steam baths, mud packs, massage, water exercise and water massage (where the water is sprayed in a fine, powerful jet on to one area of the body).

Rheumatic conditions have always been amongst the disorders treated with great success by spa therapy. Galen, a great Roman physician and a father of modern medicine, placed water therapy first on his list of practices to cure rheumatism and related complaints. Not surprisingly, the Romans were responsible for establishing many of the spas which still exist in Britain and Europe. Some of these are active and functioning as spas to this day. Most, sadly, have been closed down in the years since the Second World War.

In this country there are spas with a proud history of healing the rheumatic disorders, and more exist in Europe. Yet most of these no longer use the waters over which they are built! Instead, they use chlorinated tap water which contains none of the qualities of the healing spring water. To illustrate the variety in healing waters, here are examples of spas in Britain founded for their effects on the rheumatic disorders.

● Bath has the only natural hot springs in Britain, coming to the surface at a temperature of 120°F (49°C). These 'thermal waters' were renowned for their soothing and relaxing effect on the muscles and painful joints, and for their ability to lift one's mood. At present, there is a hospital for rheumatic diseases in Bath which, though making use of hot baths, does not use the natural hot spring waters in its scheme of treatment.

● The town of Droitwich was founded on its salt industry and, not surprisingly, its spring waters are so high in salt content as to be called brine. Droitwich was considered the strongest and most effective brine bath in the world, apart from the Dead Sea.

Poor circulation is a common and debilitating feature of many of the rheumatic diseases, which this warm brine water greatly improves. Brine also allows greater buoyancy, effectively reducing your body weight so that exercises may be performed in the water which would be painful or impossible otherwise. The result of this spa treatment is a swift improvement in strength, mobility and circulation which reinstates health, especially in those with advanced rheumatic disease.

● Woodhall Spa also supplies water with a high salt content, though nothing to compare with Droitwich. Additionally, the spring water contains iodine, which is necessary for the correct functioning of the thyroid glands. This water was therefore taken internally as well as being used for bathing. Another attraction to Woodhall was the use of mud, still containing the therapeutic qualities of the water, which was made into packs and applied to the affected joints to reduce pain and inflammation. Currently Woodhall Spa is used for rheumatic conditions, but neither the mud nor the natural spring water is used.

The spa, or health farm, provides an atmosphere of caring and supports a holistic approach to health. Great emphasis is placed on diet, rest, relaxation, and positive thinking. Most include opportunities for massage, exercise, and activities which help you to achieve renewed health and vigour. There are active spas in Britain and Europe which can treat your rheumatic disorder. Please refer to the Appendix for further details.

Saunas are a Finnish invention, used in that country to clean the body and maintain good health. They are simply small wooden huts, or rooms, which contain a stove surrounded by stones. The stones are heated and when the room reaches a suitable temperature water is poured on the stones. You sit in the sauna for 10–20 minutes, alternating the intense, moist heat with cold showers. The combination stimulates circulation, relaxes muscles and removes toxins from your body by causing perspiration. Many cases of rheumatism are eased by regular use of a sauna.

Those new to the experience, or those with diabetes or heart trouble, should take a first sauna at a temperature of 185–194°F (85°–90°C). Later, try a temperature of between 212° and 248°F (100° and 120°C). A sauna should always last for at least 10 minutes and usually no more than 20 minutes. Also, it should never be dry, but kept very humid by pouring water over the hot stones. Without this moisture, your eyes, nostrils, throat and lungs will feel dry and painful. The sauna always ends with a cold shower.

Most of the philosophies and health practices from the East are based upon the principle of opposite forces, called yin and yang, which are present in all things. These forces fluctuate in order to complement each other and establish balance. In the body, yin and yang circulate as life-force through meridians and nodes which correspond approximately with the nervous system. The life-force is also called ch'i, ki or qi. Your health is good when its circulation is unimpaired and poor when it is blocked or sluggish.

An imbalance between yin and yang creates unhealthy changes in the circulation of ch'i and some practices have been developed in the East which remedy this imbalance and enhance the circulation of life-force. These practices have, over generations of people, become a way of life and are not used only when illness becomes apparent but often on a daily basis. In the West, this is called preventative medicine and many people are now realizing the benefits and rewards of treating their health as something to be invested in and 'topped up' each day.

Eastern medicine is holistic – it considers the health of the whole person, not just the most obvious symptoms. Therefore, the whole person is treated so that health, once established, is maintained and valued through day-to-day behaviour. The following practices, although originating in the East, are becoming increasingly popular in the West. In their transition to Western cultures they have undergone some changes, if only of terminology.

These remedies may have especial effect on the following disorders:

Bursitis	Osteoarthritis
Fibrositis	Palindromic rheumatism
Gout	Psychogenic rheumatism
Infective arthritis	Rheumatoid arthritis
Juvenile rheumatoid arthritis	Sciatica
Lumbago	Spondylitis
Menopausal arthritis	Synovitis
Myositis	Tendinitis
Neuritis	Tenosynovitis

Acupuncture

Acupuncture is based on the principle of life-force as it circulates through a network of meridians and nodes, or loci, within the body. By inserting a fine metal needle into the body at one or more of these nodes, the flow of ch'i may be controlled. If you imagine each node as an intersection of roads and the needle as the traffic control lights you may understand the purpose of the needles more clearly. For, depending on the positioning of the needles, your life-force may be slowed or stimulated to improve the circulation and balance of yin and yang which results in health.

The exact location of the needles along the line of a meridian determines where in your body the benefit is felt. For instance, in treating pain it may be that the source of pain is at one location in the body, the pain itself felt in another location, and the acupuncture point to treat the pain in quite another. The acupuncturist knows how to feel the circulation of life-force through a form of pulse taking, which indicates where and how to position the needle.

It is not necessary to understand how acupuncture works in order for it be beneficial to you, just as you don't need to know how aspirin works in order for it to be effective. But because acupuncture is still a new practice in the West, you may feel more at ease in considering its use if you know more about it.

No one seems to know precisely how old the practice of acupuncture is – only that it began in the East and has been in use for thousands of years. A Dutch doctor wrote a document about acupuncture in 1683 after a visit to the Orient. This is believed to be the first written work on the subject presented in the West. From that time, Western scientists and doctors have been questioning and studying the effects of acupuncture on health. Recent times have shown perhaps the most diligent research, possibly due to the cross-cultural exchange between East and West since the Second World War.

There are thousands of 'miracle' stories told of the effects of acupuncture, ranging from pain relief to removal of all signs of disease. Often these improvements have been long term or, when the acupuncture is used repeatedly, permanent. However, a good deal of scepticism remains in the West because the scientific reason for the success of acupuncture is obscure. But today, many hospitals, doctors and medical researchers want to understand acupuncture and a great many medical studies are being undertaken around the world to measure and explain the effects of acupuncture by using it.

Acupuncture may have to wait some time before being welcomed into general medical practice, though it may reside comfortably within the GP's surgery – especially if used for the relief of chronic pain. Hopefully, as acupuncture becomes more 'normal', more doctors may choose to train in it – learning the 'map' of acupuncture points on the body as well as the philosophy of health and healing behind it.

However, many people are already taking advantage of the expertise of highly qualified acupuncturists to relieve their symptoms and to greatly improve their health. If you decide to visit an acupuncturist, please contact The Council for Acupuncture (see Appendix) to find a qualified practitioner in your area. You will probably have to pay and should anticipate an interview on your first visit. This interview will help the acupuncturist determine what sort of person you are: your mental and emotional state, your sleeping patterns, your attitudes, your food and drink preferences, and so on. This information, along with observation of you, will help him or her to place the needles correctly for maximum effectiveness.

When you receive acupuncture, the needles should enter your bare flesh so you will be asked to remove some or all of your clothing. The needles are put in place and left in position for several minutes. Use this time to think only of your health or, if you prefer, don't think – just lie there. You may experience a tingling, warmth, or any number of other sensations, including the desire to laugh. These are all part of the healing experience.

When the needles are removed, the acupuncturist will probably advise you on diet or other of your lifestyle patterns which you can change to help remedy your particular disorder. These provide a good background to the effects of the acupuncture and are usually well worth following.

The rheumatic diseases are considered part of the Bi Syndrome in Eastern medicine. That is, they are caused by an obstruction of the circulation of blood and life-force due to an 'invasion of cold and wind'. There is a high success rate in the treatment, through acupuncture, of rheumatic disorders provided the disease is treated as early as possible. Initially success is in the form of pain relief and reduction of swelling and inflammation. However, regular visits to your acupuncturist will see continued improvement in most forms of rheumatic disease – especially if you take responsibility for other aspects of your health at the same time, such as diet, rest, activity and attitude.

● A modern-day version of acupuncture is gaining in popularity in hospitals. This is the practice of stimulating the acupuncture loci with very mild electric current sent through the fine needle. It is used predominantly for anaesthesia and pain relief. In China, many types of operation are performed with this as the only, or the major, form of anaesthesia – attracting considerable interest from doctors in the West. There are no side effects from this form of anaesthesia, as there are from anaesthetic drugs, therefore it is much safer and causes no change in basic body function during the course of surgery. It is also inexpensive and post-operative recovery is more rapid.

● Just a word on hygiene, all qualified practitioners are required either to supply you with your own needles or use disposable ones.

Acupressure and Shiatzu

Acupressure and shiatzu use the same principles and the same nodes and meridians as acupuncture – but leave out the needles. Instead, pressure is exerted upon these points using a finger, knuckle or fingernail. The amount of pressure, the length of time it is held and whether it is held still or with slight movement governs the effect the acupressure has on the flow of ch'i in your body. Pressure applied firmly and deeply will stimulate the flow of ch'i, applied gently will slow it. As in acupuncture, the intention is to establish balance between yin and yang, improving health and the circulation of life-force.

Acupressure and shiatzu are virtually the same in practice. However, acupressure probably originated in China, shiatzu in Japan. Both practices have been simplified to some extent in their progress into the West.

The beauty of shiatzu and acupressure is that you may perform them yourself, upon yourself. You can learn the techniques gradually and, once you have mastered the position of the nodes, or loci, that match your ailment, you may use the pressure techniques upon yourself. Acupressure and shiatzu are used predominantly for pain relief and to prevent illness developing.

Moxibustion

Moxibustion also uses the loci of acupuncture, again without the needles. Instead, small cone-shaped twists of moxi (the 'cotton' from wormwood, a type of herb) are ignited and placed over the acupuncture points. The moxi smoulders and is removed before it contacts the skin. The heat which results from moxibustion acts upon the flow of ch'i in a similar way to acupuncture. In Eastern medicine, rheumatism is caused by the Bi Syndrome – an invasion of cold and wind. Moxibustion sounds the perfect antagonist to Bi, as though it could heat it right out of your body!

As you might suspect, moxibustion hasn't the same popularity that acupuncture and acupressure enjoy in the West, yet it is effective in the same way. It is probable that moxibustion was introduced, centuries ago, to answer the social and religious demands of some Eastern cultures. For these cultures, any treatment given to improve health had to be non-invasive. That is, it had to act upon the body without intruding upon it in any way – even to the exclusion of using the delicate needles of acupuncture. Moxibustion produces at most a slight, temporary redness on the surface of the skin and therefore does not 'invade' the body. Your acupuncturist may use this technique for some treatment; it is not a remedy which you should perform upon yourself.

Reflexology and Ear Acupuncture

In Eastern medicine, the ears, hands and feet are sometimes called homunculi, that is, they are considered to be small models of the human being. Of course, they don't resemble the shape of the human body, but there are points on each of them which correspond to all of the body's organs, glands, joints and so on. Massage, acupuncture or acupressure may be performed on these points to stimulate the areas of body they relate to and, as in all Eastern medicine, the intention is to establish health through balance and the free circulation of life-force.

● Hand and foot reflexology have been practised in some form for centuries and in many different cultures. Ancient European, African and Egyptian as well as Oriental peoples divided the body into zones or regions and confined treatment of disease to the zone in which it appeared. The number of zones and their exact placement has, of course, varied from culture to culture. The general placement has remained the same, however, as have the benefits derived from stimulation of the reflex points.

You may perform reflexology upon yourself – it is especially easy when using reflex points on the hand. However, it is a very soothing experience to receive the treatment from someone else and the more experienced they are in giving it, the better its effects on you. In any case, reflexology is not harmful. There are only a few points to observe for the sake of safety and comfort:

● Apply only light pressure when pressing against a bone that is near to the surface.

● Avoid deep or prolonged stimulation of a point when pregnancy or heart disease is indicated.

● A little done often is better than a lot done all at once.

If you choose to be treated through reflexology, it is likely that your feet will be the source of the reflexologist's attention. They are slightly more sensitive to treatment than the hands. You will be asked to sit in a very comfortable chair, usually a reclining one, with your feet raised and your knees slightly bent. The reflexologist will sit facing the soles of your feet.

A little talc may be rubbed over your feet and the reflexologist will begin to massage. However wonderful this may feel to you, the reflexologist is working hard to learn about your state of health by how you respond to pressure on the reflex points on your feet. For instance, you may flinch or pull a face when one or more points are pressed and these reactions are noted by the reflexologist.

When the initial massage has been completed (you will probably feel wonderfully relaxed) the reflexologist will go back to those reflex points which were noticeably tender to you. These points correspond to areas of your body which are not well. The reflexologist will stimulate these points according to the degree of discomfort you feel. If you feel a lot, the stimulation will be mild; if you only feel slight discomfort, the pressure may be increased to stimulate these areas more.

This treatment is repeated often over a period of days or weeks and then on a regular basis to maintain health. It may be used safely with other forms of treatment, both natural and drug-based. Because it deals with body zones, reflexology will not confine itself to one joint, for instance, but will improve your health in several ways. You may find your digestion improves as well as the pain in your knees!

● The ear is also a homunculus – a small model of the human body. There is a point on the ear for every part of the body and these points may be stimulated through acupuncture or acupressure to improve health. Because the ear has fairly tight and inaccessible curves and corners, it is usually necessary to go to an acupuncturist in order to receive this treatment. Recently, however, practitioners have learned to insert small studs into the acupuncture points so that the patients may subsequently simply press the studs themselves to receive the benefits of the treatment. This is being used successfully for pain relief, obesity, smoking and chronic ailments. Acupuncture anaesthesia may be performed by stimulating points on the ear and the body at the same time. Today, this is usually done with mild electrical current passed through the needles.

The rheumatic disorders are readily eased by these treatments, both in terms of pain relief and improved muscle and joint function.

Appendix

FURTHER READING* AND USEFUL NAMES & ADDRESSES

CHAPTER 1:
Arthritis Care: 6 Grosvenor Crescent, London SW1X 7ER, tel. 01–235–0902/5

The National Osteoporosis Society: PO Box 10, Barton Meade House, Radstock, Bath BA3 3YB, tel. (0761) 32472

Back Pain Association: Grundy House, 31–33 Park Road, Teddington, Middlesex TW11 0AB, tel. 01–977–5474/5

British Medical Association: BMA House, Tavistock Square, London WC1H 9JP, tel. 01–387–4499

Rheumatic Diseases, by S. L. Kumar, World Homoeopathic Links, New Delhi, India, 1982

Overcoming The Menopause Naturally, Dr Caroline Shreeve, Century Arrow, 1986

CHAPTER 2:
Making the Most of Your Doctor, Dr Jennifer King, Dr David Pendleton and Dr Peter Tate, Thames Methuen, 1985

CHAPTER 3:
British Holistic Medical Association: 170 Gloucester Place, London NW1 6DX, tel. 01–262–5299

The Natural Medicines Society: Edith Lewis House, Back Lane, Ilkeston, Derbyshire DE7 8EJ

Institute for Complementary Medicine: 21 Portland Place, London W1N 3AF, tel. 01–631–4368

The Institute for Complementary Medicine Yearbook, compiled by Jane Foulkes, W. Foulsham & Co. Ltd, 1987 (This contains a very thorough listing of national and regional contact names and addresses for most of the natural therapies, as well as guidelines to recognizing qualified practitioners.)

CHAPTER 4:
Action Against Allergy (AAA): 43 The Downs, London SW20 8HG, tel. 01–947–5082

National Society for Research into Allergy: PO Box 45, Hinkley, Leicestershire LE10 1JY

The Vegan Society: 33–35 George Street, Oxford OX1 2AX (please send a s.a.e. for membership details)

Allergies Your Hidden Enemy, Theron G. Randolph MD & Ralph W. Moss Ph.D., Turnstone Press Ltd, 1980

Arthritic Cookbook, Mary Caver & Margaret Smith, Hamlyn, 1984

About Raw Juices, John B. Lust, Thorsons Publishers Ltd, 1977

Nutritional Medicine, Dr Stephen Davies & Dr Alan Stewart, Pan Books, 1987

Zen Macrobiotics, Georges Ohsawa, The Ohsawa Foundation, 1965

Why You Don't Need Meat, Peter Cox, Thorsons Publishers, 1986

The Vegetarian Epicure, Anna Thomas, Penguin Books Limited, 1974

Arthritis & Folk Medicine, D. C. Jarvis MD, Pan Books, 1960

Hanssen's Complete Cider Vinegar, Maurice Hanssen, Thorsons Publishers Ltd, 1974

CHAPTER 5: Extend: Mrs Penny Copple, Director of Development, 5 Conway Road, Sheringham, Norfolk NR26 8DD

The Keep Fit Association: The National Secretary, 16 Upper Woburn Place, London WC1H 0QG, tel. 01–387–4349

The Women's League of Health & Beauty: 18 Charing Cross Road, London WC2 0HR, tel. 01–240–8456

British Wheel of Yoga: 80 Leckhampton Road, Cheltenham, Gloucestershire GL53 0BN

Buster Crabbe's Arthritis Exercise Book, Buster Crabbe, Angus & Robertson (UK) Ltd, 1980

CHAPTER 6: British College of Naturopathy and Osteopathy: Frazer House, 6 Netherhall Gardens, London NW3 5RR, tel. 01–435–7830

British School of Osteopathy: 1–4 Suffolk Street, London SW1Y 4HG, tel. 01–839–2060

The College of Osteopaths: Administrative Services, 110 Thorkhill Road, Thames Ditton, Surrey KT7 0UW, tel. 01–398–3308

European School of Osteopathy: 104 Tonbridge Road, Maidstone, Kent ME16 8SL, tel. (0622) 671558

British Chiropractic Association: 5 First Avenue, Chelmsford, Essex CM1 1RX, tel. (0245) 358487

The Institute of Pure Chiropractic: PO Box 126, Oxford OX1 1UF, tel. (0865) 246687

Northern Institute of Massage: 100 Waterloo Road, Blackpool, Lancashire FY4 1AW, tel. (0253) 403548

Shiatzu Society: 19 Langside Park, Kilbarchan, Strathclyde PA10 2EP, tel. (05057) 4657

West London School of Therapeutic Massage: 41 St Luke's Road, London W11 1DD, tel. 01–229–7411

Chiropractic For Everyone, Anthea Courtenay, Penguin Books Limited, 1987

Self-Massage, Monika Struna with Connie Church, Century Hutchinson Ltd, 1983

Osteopathy, Edward Triance DO, Thorsons Publishers Ltd, 1986

Mind Your Body, E. H. Shattock, Turnstone Press Ltd, 1979

Relaxation & Meditation Techniques, Leon Chaitow, Thorsons Publishers Ltd, 1983

Naturopathic Medicine, Roger Newman Turner, Thorsons Publishers Ltd, 1984

Your Complete Stress-Proofing Programme, Leon Chaitow, Thorsons Publishers Ltd, 1983

Self Help For Your Nerves, Dr Claire Weekes, Angus & Robertson (UK) Ltd, 1962

CHAPTER 7: British Homoeopathic Association: 27a Devonshire Street, London W1N 1RJ, tel. 01–935–2163

A Guide To Biochemic Tissue Salts, Dr Andrew Stanway, Van Dyke Books, 1982

Homoeopathy For Everyone, Drs Sheila & Robin Gibson Penguin Books Limited, 1987

Biochemic Handbook, revised by a homoeopathic physician, New Era Laboratories Ltd, 1975

CHAPTER 8: National Institute of Medical Herbalists: 41 Hatherley Road, Winchester, Hampshire SO22 6RR

Comfrey: Supplied by The Henry Doubleday Research Association, Convent Lane, Bocking, Braintree, Essex CM7 6RW

The Dr Edward Bach Healing Centre: 'Mount Vernon', Sotwell, Wallingford, Oxfordshire OX10 0PZ

Practical Aromatherapy, Shirley Price, Thorsons Publishers Ltd, 1983

Aromatherapy Handbook, Daniele Ryman, Century Hutchinson Ltd, 1984

Aromatherapy, Raymond Lautie & Andre Passebecq, Thorsons Publishers Ltd, 1979

The Home Herbal, Barbara Griggs, Pan Books, 1982

Bach Flower Therapy, Mechthild Scheffer, Thorsons Publishers Ltd, 1986

Edward Bach Physician, Nora Weeks, C. W. Daniel Co. Ltd, 1983

CHAPTER 9: *Crystal Healing*, Edmund Harold, Aquarian Press, 1986

Crystals: supplied by R. G. Bonewitz, 10 South Molton Street, London W1Y 1DF, tel. 01–499–0017

CHAPTER 10: *Spas That Heal*, William A. R. Thomson, A. & C. Black (Publishers) Ltd, 1978

Practical Hydrotherapy, Gerhard Leibold, Thorsons Publishers Ltd, 1980

My Water Cure, Sebastian Kneipp, Thorsons Publishers Ltd, 1979

Sauna For Health, Donald Law, Godfrey Cave, 1978

CHAPTER 11: British Reflexology Association: 12 Pond Road, London SE3 9JL, tel. 01–852–6062

Bayly School of Reflexology: Monks Orchard, Whitbourne, Worcester WR6 5RB, tel. Knightwick (0886) 21207

The Council for Acupuncture: 11 Albany Road, Stratford-upon-Avon, Warwickshire CV37 6PG

Is Acupuncture For You? J. R. Worsley, Element Books Ltd, 1985

Acupressure Techniques: A Self-Help Guide, Dr Julian Kenyon, Thorsons Publishers Ltd, 1987

Hand & Foot Reflexology: A Self Help Guide, Kevin & Barbara Kunz, Prentice Hall, 1984

GLOSSARY

Acute: short, sharp and severe symptoms or phase of your disease

Assimilate: to absorb or transform a food, drug or other substance

Atrophy: to waste away or diminish in size

Chronic: persisting and recurring over a long period of time

Density: as in bone, the quantity of tissue in a compact area

Diuretic: that which increases the passing of urine

Endocrine: as in system, secretes hormones into your blood and lymph

Hormone: a substance which regulates the activity of a specific organ

Lymph: a liquid, made from the fluids which surround all your body's tissues, which helps in the transportation of nutrients and toxins

Metabolism: the grand total of all the processes which keep you alive!

Placebo: a substance with no real medicinal value, but a symbolic drug

Rarefaction: as in bone, losing density and weight, but not losing size